A Clinical Guide to Pediatric Sleep
Diagnosis and Management of Sleep Problems

A Clinical Guide to Pediatric Sleep
Diagnosis and Management of Sleep Problems

Jodi A. Mindell, Ph.D.
Saint Joseph's University
Children's Hospital of Philadelphia
Philadelphia, Pennsylvania

Judith A. Owens, M.D., M.P.H.
Brown University Medical School
Hasbro Children's Hospital
Providence, Rhode Island

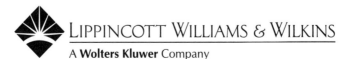

LIPPINCOTT WILLIAMS & WILKINS
A **Wolters Kluwer** Company

Philadelphia · Baltimore · New York · London
Buenos Aires · Hong Kong · Sydney · Tokyo

Acquisitions Editor: Timothy Y. Hiscock
Developmental Editor: Nicole T. Wagner
Production Editor: Emily Lerman
Manufacturing Manager: Colin J. Warnock
Cover Designer: J. Norton
Compositor: Lippincott Williams & Wilkins Desktop Division
Printer: Victor Graphics

Library of Congress Cataloging-in-Publication Data

Mindell, Jodi A.
  A clinical guide to pediatric sleep : diagnosis and management of sleep problems /
Jodi A. Mindell, Judith A. Owens.
    p. ; cm.
  Includes bibliographic references and index.
  ISBN-13 978-0-7817-4012-8 (alk. paper)
  ISBN-10 0-7817-4012-6 (alk. paper)
    1. Sleep disorders in chidren. 2. Children—health and hygiene. 3. Sleep. I. Owens,
Judith A. II. Title.
    [DNLM: 1. Sleep Disorders—diagnosis—Adolescence. 2. Sleep
Disorders—diagnosis—Child. 3. Sleep Disorders—therapy—Adolescence. 4. Sleep
Disorders—therapy—Child. WM 188 M663c 2003]
  RJ506.5.S55 M54 2003
  618.92′8498—dc21
                                                                        2002040954

Care has been taken to confirm the accuracy of the information presented and to describe
generally accepted practices. However, the authors and publisher are not responsible for
errors or omissions or for any consequences from application of the information in this
book and make no warranty, expressed or implied, with respect to the currency, complete-
ness, or accuracy of the contents of the publication. Application of this information in a
particular situation remains the professional responsibility of the practitioner.

The authors and publisher have exerted every effort to ensure that drug selection and
dosage set forth in this text are in accordance with current recommendations and practice
at the time of publication. However, in view of ongoing research, changes in government
regulations, and the constant flow of information relating to drug therapy and drug reactions, the reader is urged to check the package insert for each drug for any change in indications and dosage and for added warnings and precautions. This is particularly important
when the recommended agent is a new or infrequently employed drug.

Some drugs and medical devices presented in this publication have Food and Drug
Administration (FDA) clearance for limited use in restricted research settings. It is the
responsibility of the health care provider to ascertain the FDA status of each drug or device
planned for use in their clinical practice.

10 9 8 7 6 5 4 3 2

To Scott and Caelie—JAM
To Evan and Grace—JAO

Contents

Section III: Sleep and Medications

Section IV: Sleep in Special Populations

Appendices

Preface

There are few pediatric health issues that are more common or have a more significant impact on health and well-being than childhood sleep disorders. Approximately 25% of all children experience some type of sleep problem, ranging from difficulty falling asleep and nightwakings to more serious primary sleep disorders such as sleep apnea or narcolepsy. Upwards of one-third of elementary school-aged children and 40% of adolescents have significant sleep complaints. The consequences of sleep disorders in children are serious, and range from cardiovascular problems and failure to thrive to significant behavioral concerns and academic failure. Furthermore, sleep disorders in children and adolescents are particularly important to recognize and diagnose since many of these disorders are treatable with highly effective medical and behavioral interventions.

The goal of *A Clinical Guide to Pediatric Sleep: Diagnosis and Management of Sleep Problems* is to provide pediatricians and other pediatric health care providers with the information they need to recognize, evaluate, and treat sleep issues in children and adolescents. *A Clinical Guide to Pediatric Sleep* synthesizes current state-of-the-art information about the assessment and treatment of sleep disorders in children and adolescents and provides a comprehensive but accessible resource for practitioners.

A Clinical Guide to Pediatric Sleep is divided into four sections, with an extensive appendix of parenting handouts for health care practitioners to use in their practice.

Section I addresses basic sleep issues in pediatric practice, including information on screening and prevention of sleep problems, basic principles of healthy sleep in children and adolescents, and an overview of the impact of sleep problems on children and families. It also provides an overview of sleep biology and basic information about sleep diagnostic tools, including polysomnography. Finally, this section presents information on developmental aspects of sleep, including normal sleep parameters and commonly experienced sleep problems for each age group.

Section II provides comprehensive information on evaluation, treatment, management, and prognosis for each of the most common pediatric sleep disorders. This section also contains symptom-based algorithms based on the three most common presentations of sleep problems in the clinical setting: difficulty falling asleep, nightwakings, and daytime sleepiness. Because there are multiple sleep problems that can account for each of these presenting symptoms, the algorithms enable the health care provider to evaluate sleep complaints in a stepwise fashion with the goal of developing the most appropriate treatment plan.

Section III discusses medications and sleep, both those medications that affect sleep and those medications that may be prescribed for sleep problems.

Section IV presents information on sleep problems in special populations, including developmentally disabled children and pediatric patients who have a comorbid medical or psychiatric problem.

Finally, a highly comprehensive *Appendix* provides resources for pediatric providers, including intake and screening questionnaires and parent education handouts for each age group and each sleep disorder. A national listing of clinical resources and other informational resources (e.g., foundations, internet sites) is also included.

Our hope is that this book will provide every pediatric practitioner with a comprehensive resource on pediatric sleep, so that all children and their families can get the sleep they need.

Acknowledgments

No project of this magnitude is ever developed without the enthusiasm and support of others. We extend our thanks not only to the following individuals who supported this particular work, but to the families who shared their experiences (and sleepless nights!) to help further our knowledge of pediatric sleep.

Great appreciation goes to those who provided their input into this project, including Dr. Lisa Meltzer, Dr. Alex Mason, Dr. Carol Rosen, and Dr. Manisha Whitman. Additionally, a big thank you to Clare McAneny for her incredible secretarial support and much appreciation to Joanne Elliott for providing the polysomnography records.

Finally, our deepest appreciation to those who have supported this project: Timothy Y. Hiscock of Lippincott Williams & Wilkins for his enthusiasm from the very beginning; Nicole Wagner, developmental editor, and Emily Lerman, production editor, who shepherded this book through the publishing process; and Claudia Schmidt, Gordon Rawlinson, and Kathleen Dittman of Johnson's Baby who have embraced sleep education as being a priority for every family.

And, most importantly, to our families for their unwavering support, enthusiasm, and patience.

A Clinical Guide to Pediatric Sleep
Diagnosis and Management of Sleep Problems

1

Sleep in the Pediatric Practice

It is estimated that by the age of 2 years the average child has spent about 9,500 hours (or a total of 13 months) sleeping, in contrast to 8,000 hours for all waking activities combined. Sleep is *the* primary activity of the brain during early development. Between the ages of 2 and 5 years, children spend equal amounts of time awake and asleep. And throughout childhood and adolescence, sleep continues to account for about 40% of a child's average day.

While sleep clearly occupies a major portion of the childhood years, childhood *sleeplessness*, in its many forms, clearly constitutes a major parental (and therefore, health care practitioner) concern. Inadequate, disrupted, poor-quality, nonrestful, and at times elusive sleep constitute one of the most common complaints raised by parents to pediatricians and pediatric practitioners. In contrast, the relationship between *insufficient or disturbed sleep* and the many manifestations of *sleepiness* is less frequently recognized by parents, but is nonetheless a major contributor to mood, behavior, academic, and health problems in childhood. As such, daytime sleepiness also becomes an important issue on many levels for the health care provider to recognize and address.

However, given the expanding number of competing demands for increasingly smaller amounts of time and the information overload that the average busy pediatric practitioner faces on a daily basis, sleep issues in clinical practice may not always receive the attention that they deserve. The purpose of this book, therefore, is twofold: (a) to provide the practitioner with an appreciation for the pervasive impact that sleep, sleeplessness, and sleepiness have on children's and families' lives and the multiple ways in which that impact is felt in clinical pediatric practice and (b) to provide the basic knowledge and practical tools with which to approach and solve sleep problems in children and adolescents. This chapter begins to address these goals by outlining the key sleep-related issues relevant to the pediatric practitioner and by providing a general rationale and framework for integrating sleep into clinical pediatric practice.

THE TOP TEN REASONS PEDIATRIC PRACTITIONERS SHOULD CARE ABOUT SLEEP

(1) Sleep problems are common in children and adolescents. There are few pediatric health issues that are more common than childhood sleep disorders. Approximately 25% of all children experience some type of sleep problem at some point during childhood, ranging from short-term difficulties in falling asleep and nightwakings, to more serious primary sleep disorders such as obstructive sleep apnea or narcolepsy. For example, snoring, the most common symptom of sleep-disordered breathing, has a prevalence of 3% to 12% in preschool-aged children, and obstructive sleep apnea syndrome is conservatively estimated to affect 1% to 3% of the pediatric population. Other studies have reported an overall prevalence of a variety of parent-reported sleep problems ranging from 25% to 50% in preschool-aged samples to 37% in a community sample of 4- to 10-year-olds. Upward of 40% of adolescents also have significant sleep complaints. Epidemiologic studies have suggested that sleep problems in children are becoming more common; for example, the percentage of adolescents experiencing chronic insufficient sleep has risen significantly in the past few decades.

(2) Childhood sleep problems are chronic. Although many sleep problems in infants and children are transient and self-limited, the common wisdom that children "grow out of" sleep problems is not an accurate perception. Certain intrinsic and extrinsic risk factors (e.g., difficult temperament, chronic illness, neurodevelopmental delays, maternal depression, family stress) may predispose a given child to develop a more chronic sleep disturbance. A number of studies also have documented the persistence of infant sleep problems into early childhood. Some sleep problems, such as obstructive sleep apnea and some forms of insomnia, may persist into or resurface in adulthood, whereas other lifelong disorders, such as restless legs syndrome and narcolepsy, may first be identified in childhood or adolescence. Thus, early identification and treatment of these sleep disorders in the pediatric population potentially impacts on their natural history.

(3) Pediatric sleep disorders are treatable. Many highly effective medical and behavioral interventions for sleep disorders are available. The efficacy of specific behavioral interventions for nightwakings, for example, has been well documented in multiple controlled studies. In addition, new treatments for sleep disorders, as well as empirical testing of existing treatments, are being actively pursued. Furthermore, children who have been successfully treated for sleep problems (e.g., adenotonsillectomy for obstructive sleep apnea) show marked improvements in mood, behavior, attention, and academic performance. Because at least some of the significant effects of sleep disturbances in children appear to be reversible, recognition and treatment of sleep problems by primary health care providers offers an important opportunity for secondary, as well as for primary prevention.

(4) Sleep problems are preventable. Not only are sleep problems treatable, but they are highly preventable. The pediatric visit is an opportunity to educate parents about normal sleep in children and to teach them strategies to prevent sleep problems from either developing in the first place (primary prevention) or becoming chronic when problems already exist (secondary prevention). Effective preventative measures (see Chapter 3) may include educating parents of newborns about normal sleep durations and patterns, suggesting that parents put their 3- to 6-month-old infant to bed "drowsy but awake" in order to avoid dependence on parental presence at sleep onset and to foster the infant's ability to "self-soothe" and discussing the importance of regular bedtimes, bedtime routines, and transitional objects for toddlers. Older children and their parents can be provided with basic information about good "sleep hygiene" (Appendices F15 and F16) and adequate sleep amounts.

(5) Sleep problems in children have a major impact on the family. Sleep problems are a significant source of distress for families and may be one of the primary reasons for caregiver stress in families with children who have chronic illnesses or handicapping conditions, such as severe neurodevelopmental delays. Furthermore, the impact of childhood sleep problems is intensified by their direct effect on parents' sleep, resulting in daytime fatigue, mood disturbances, and a decreased level of effective parenting. Poor sleep has even been implicated as a risk factor for child physical abuse. Conversely, successful intervention by the health care practitioner not only helps parents develop behavioral strategies that may generalize for use with daytime behavior problems, but has the effect of improving the sleep of the entire family.

(6) Sleep problems constitute one of the most common parental complaints. Given that sleep problems have such a significant impact on both children and their families, sleep concerns are very common parental complaints in pediatric practices. One study of practicing pediatricians noted that 23% of their patients between the ages of 6 months and 4 years experienced sleep problems that were brought to the attention of the physician. Sleep concerns were ranked as the fifth leading concern of parents, following illness, feeding problems, behavior problems, and physical abnormalities. It was also noted that parents were more concerned about sleep problems than difficulties with language development, motor development, toileting, and teething.

(7) Sleep is necessary for children's optimal functioning. A wealth of empirical evidence, much of it gathered in the past decade, clearly indicates that children and adolescents experience significant daytime sleepiness as a result of inadequate or disturbed sleep and that significant performance impairments and mood dysfunction are associated with that daytime sleepiness. The evidence comes from several lines of research, including studies of children under conditions of restricted sleep in the laboratory setting, assessment of functional impairment in children identified as "poor sleepers" or with sleep disorders such as obstructive sleep apnea, and documentation of sleep quality and quantity in children identified with primary mood, behavioral, and/or academic performance dysfunction such as attention deficit-hyperactivity disorder (ADHD).

Increased physiologic sleepiness in children following experimental sleep restriction (e.g., 6.5 hours per night for 7 nights) has been associated with oppositional and inattentive behavior, evidence of impaired verbal fluency and creativity, and impaired abstract problem solving, as well as decreased speed and efficiency in the completion of tasks. In a number of other studies, although not all, infants, toddlers, and schoolchildren characterized as poor sleepers have an increased prevalence and severity of parent- and teacher-reported behavioral difficulties and mood problems in comparison to children without sleep problems. In addition, children with obstructive sleep apnea have significant academic performance deficits. Conversely, children with academic and behavioral problems are more likely to have symptoms of sleep-disordered breathing (loud snoring) and to have symptoms of restless legs syndrome/periodic limb movement disorder. Poor academic performance also is associated with sleep problems and insufficient sleep in adolescents and college students. Although such variables as individual differences in the type and degree of functional impairment and the degree of sleep disturbance required to produce impairments have yet to be described, it is clear that poor sleep and poor outcomes in children and adolescents frequently go hand in hand.

(8) Sleep affects every aspect of a child's physical, emotional, cognitive, and social development. We are just beginning to understand the negative consequences of inadequate or poor sleep in children on a host of developmental domains, including mood, behavior, and learning, as well as on health outcomes. Mood problems in children with sleep disturbances are virtually universal, particularly exacerbation of negative mood and, equally importantly, a decrease in positive mood or affect. Regulation of mood, or the use of cognitive strategies to modulate and guide emotions, also appears to be affected by sleep quality and quantity; thus, chronic poor sleep during critical periods of development of affective regulation may have long-term consequences on emotional health. Behavioral responses to sleepiness in children, although highly variable, may be broadly described as manifestations of dysregulation of arousal, impairment of attention, and failure to inhibit inappropriate behavioral responses (poor impulse control). These impairments in both mood regulation and impulse control have obvious implications for the development of a child's ability to successfully negotiate social interactions with family and peers.

Higher-level cognitive functions, such as cognitive flexibility and the ability to reason and think abstractly, appear to be most consistently sensitive to the effects of disturbed or insufficient sleep. Other neuropsychological domains, such as attention and memory, also demonstrate significant impairments, although these appear to require longer periods and higher levels of sleep restriction or disruption. Finally, health outcomes of inadequate sleep include an increase in accidental injuries (ranging from minor injuries to drowsy driving–related motor vehicle fatalities) and potential deleterious effects on the cardiovascular, immune, and various metabolic systems, including glucose metabolism and endocrine function.

(9) The coexistence of sleep problems exacerbates virtually all medical, psychiatric, developmental, and psychosocial problems in childhood. Because of the multiple manifestations of poor and insufficient sleep, the clinical symptoms of any primary medical or psychiatric disorder are likely to be worsened by comorbid sleep problems. Furthermore, sleep problems themselves tend to be more common in those children and adolescents with chronic medical and psychiatric conditions. Thus, attentional and academic dysfunction in ADHD is likely to be more severe, mood disturbances like depression in adolescents become worse, chronic pain conditions like juvenile rheumatoid arthritis are exacerbated, and parent–child conflicts are often more problematic in the setting of poor sleep. Conversely, improving sleep has the benefit of improving clinical outcome as well.

Vulnerable populations, such as children who are at high risk for developmental and behavioral problems because of poverty, parental substance abuse and mental illness, or violence in the home, may be even more likely to experience "double jeopardy" as a result of sleep problems. In other words, not only are these children at higher risk for *developing* sleep problems as a result of such conditions as chaotic home environments, chronic medical issues like iron deficiency anemia, and neglect, they are also less likely to be *diagnosed* with sleep problems because of limited access to health care services. Finally, they are likely to suffer more serious *consequences* from those sleep problems than their less vulnerable peers.

(10) Sleep is a public health issue. While pediatricians have become more vigilant in monitoring and providing education about virtually every aspect of children's health and well-being (such as television viewing habits, substance abuse prevention, and parental disciplinary style), recent surveys suggest that sleep issues in pediatric practice are frequently inadequately addressed. In a recent survey of over 600 community-based pediatricians, more than 20% of the respondents did not routinely screen for sleep problems in school-aged children in the context of the well-child visit, only about 25% routinely screened toddlers and preschoolers for snoring, and less than 40% questioned adolescents about their sleep habits, despite the respondents' acknowledgment of the importance of sleep in health, behavior, and school performance. Studies suggest that physicians are not adequately trained in sleep medicine during medical school and residency and that very little time in the curriculum is devoted to pediatric sleep issues. However, in a recent survey of inner-city preadolescents, the students themselves identified their health care provider as one of the most important and reliable sources of information about healthy sleep; this suggests a need for pediatric health care providers to become more involved in this aspect of health guidance, particularly because schools seldom provide any health education regarding the development of healthy sleep habits.

Finally, from a public health perspective, the financial burden of childhood sleep problems is considerable. For example, it has been estimated that the economic cost of health professional contacts for infant crying and sleeping problems is the equivalent of 104 million U.S. dollars per annum. A recent study documented a 226% increase in health care utilization, including hospital days, drugs, and emergency department visits, in children with obstructive sleep apnea; furthermore, the percentage of hospital discharges in the United States related to obesity-associated sleep apnea in youths aged 6 to 17 years increased fivefold from 1979 to 1999.

CONCEPTUAL FRAMEWORK OF SLEEP DISTURBANCES IN CHILDREN

Basic Mechanisms

Most sleep problems in children may be broadly conceptualized as involving one or more basic mechanisms: inadequate duration of sleep for age (*insufficient sleep quantity*), disruption and fragmentation of sleep (*poor sleep quality*), or *inappropriate timing of the sleep period* (as occurs in circadian rhythm disturbances). Insufficient sleep is usually the result of difficulty initiating (delayed sleep onset) and/or maintaining sleep (prolonged nightwakings), whereas sleep fragmentation most often results from frequent, repetitive, and brief arousals during sleep. Inadequate sleep duration, especially in older children and adolescents, may also represent a conscious lifestyle decision to sacrifice sleep in favor of competing priorities, such as homework and social activities (Fig.1.1).

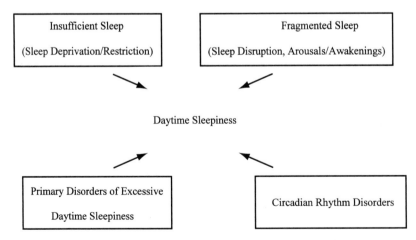

FIG. 1.1. Basic mechanisms of sleep disturbances in children.

Etiology: Is It Behavioral or Physiologic?

The underlying cause of insufficient sleep or poor sleep quality may be related to *behavioral factors* (e.g., bedtime resistance resulting in shortened sleep duration); *medical factors* (e.g., obstructive sleep apnea causing frequent brief arousals); or in many cases both factors. Successful intervention is predicated on identifying these factors.

Sleep as an Intrinsic Biological Process/Sleep as a Learned Behavior

Despite their seemingly contradictory nature, it is important for the pediatric practitioner to understand the implications of both of these concepts in approaching sleep and sleep problems in children. Few clinical paradigms in pediatrics are a better example of the need for a biopsychosocial approach than sleep. While our scientific understanding of the structure, organization, regulation, and development of sleep has exploded in the past decade and has included major advances in the genetics and neurobiology of sleep, it is clear that sleep is also impacted on by multiple psychosocial factors, ranging from exposure to environmental toxins such as lead, to cultural variables such as co-sleeping practices, and to community standards such as school start times. While much of the chronobiological "hard-wiring" of sleep is immutable, the plasticity of the developing brain makes it likely that sleep and its relationship to other neural systems in the brain are relatively more susceptible to environmental influences. Furthermore, the construct that much of sleep behavior is learned behavior not only underscores the importance of developing health-promoting sleep behaviors early in childhood but also emphasizes the role that parents and caregivers play in shaping and modifying sleep behaviors in their children.

Cultural and Family Context

It is also important to consider the cultural and family context within which sleep problems in children occur. For example, *co-sleeping* of infants and parents is a common and accepted practice in many ethnic groups, including African Americans, Hispanics, and Southeast Asians. Therefore, the goal of independent self-soothing in young infants may not be shared by these families. On the other hand, the institution of co-sleeping by parents as an attempt to address a child's underlying sleep problem ("reactive" co-sleeping) rather than as a lifestyle choice is likely to yield only a temporary respite from the problem and may set the stage for more significant and chronic sleep disturbances in children. The relative importance of sleep as a health behavior, the interpretation of problematic versus normal sleep by parents, sleeping arrangements, and the relative acceptability of various treatment strategies (e.g., the "cry it out" approach) for sleep problems are just a few additional examples of sleep issues that are influenced by cultural and family values and practices.

Impact on Functioning

As in adults, both insufficient quantity and poor quality of sleep in children usually result in excessive daytime sleepiness and decreased daytime alertness levels. However, it is important to note that sleepiness in children may not be immediately recognizable as drowsiness, yawning, and the other "classic" manifestations of sleepiness that occur in adults. Instead, as noted above, sleepiness often takes the form of mood disturbances, behavioral problems such as hyperactivity and poor impulse control, and neurocognitive dysfunctions, including inattention and impaired vigilance, that may ultimately result in significant social, school, and learning problems (Fig. 1.2).

Impact of Insufficient Sleep

- **Mood:** irritability, moodiness, poor emotional regulation
- **Cognitive functioning:** inattention, poor concentration, decreased reaction time, impaired vigilance, decreased executive functioning (decision making, problem solving), learning problems, poor academic performance
- **Behavior:** overactivity, noncompliance, oppositional behavior, poor impulse control, increased risk taking, drowsy driving
- **Family disruption:** negative impact on parents, family stress, marital discord, social problems

---

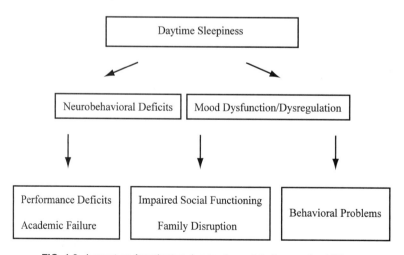

FIG. 1.2. Impact on functioning due to sleep disturbances in children.

CLASSIFICATION OF PEDIATRIC SLEEP DISORDERS

Sleep problems may be viewed as occurring along a severity and chronicity continuum that ranges from a transient and self-limited disturbance to a disorder that meets specific diagnostic criteria as outlined in the *International Classification of Sleep Disorders* (ICSD) and/or the *Diagnostic and Statistical Manual of Mental Disorders*, 4th edition (DSM-IV). It should be kept in mind that the description of the sleep problem is often quite subjective and highly dependent on parents' awareness of, expectations for, tolerance of, and interpretation of the sleep behaviors. On the other hand, as is also the case with other behavioral problems in childhood, practitioners should recognize the validity of parental concerns and opinions regarding their child's sleep patterns and behaviors. Furthermore, successful treatment of pediatric sleep problems is highly dependent on identification of parental concerns, clarification of mutually acceptable treatment goals, active exploration of opportunities and obstacles, and ongoing communication about issues and concerns.

SCREENING

The above discussion reinforces the critical need for pediatricians and primary health care providers to both screen for and recognize the symptoms of sleep disorders in children and adolescents. Pediatricians are in an ideal position to identify sleep concerns because of their regular access to children and families during well-child encounters, especially prior to school entry, and because of the inherently biopsychosocial orientation of pediatric practice. Early detection of sleep problems in children necessitates a *system* for age-appropriate screening and surveillance of pediatric populations. Developmentally appropriate screening for sleep disturbances should take place in the context of every well-child visit and the screening process should elicit parental feedback about a range of potential sleep problems. In addition, because parents may not always be aware of sleep problems, especially in older children and adolescents, it is also important to question the child directly. One simple sleep screening algorithm, the "BEARS," is outlined in Table 1.1. This five-question screening tool for pediatric sleep problems has been shown to yield significantly more information about sleep in general and about specific sleep domains than the use of a standard single question (e.g., "Does your child have any sleep problems?"). It also increases the likelihood of identifying sleep problems in the primary care setting (see Chapter 4 for a complete discussion on evaluation of pediatric sleep disorders). In addition, screening questionnaires for obstructive sleep apnea and restless legs syndrome are provided in Appendices C and D.

Furthermore, an assessment of sleep patterns and possible sleep problems should be part of the evaluation of every child presenting with behavioral and/or academic problems, especially ADHD, and with other high-risk populations, such as children with neurodevelopmental conditions, chronic medical illnesses, and genetic syndromes. Targeted screening for and surveillance of sleep problems in the pediatric practice setting is essential with these populations.

TABLE 1.1. *BEARS sleep screening algorithm*

The "BEARS" instrument is divided into five major sleep domains, providing a comprehensive screen for the major sleep disorders affecting children in the 2- to 18-year old range. Each sleep domain has a set of age-appropriate "trigger questions" for use in the clinical interview.

B = bedtime problems
E = excessive daytime sleepiness
A = awakenings during the night
R = regularity and duration of sleep
S = snoring

Examples of developmentally appropriate trigger questions:

	Toddler/preschool (2–5 years)	School-aged (6–12 years)	Adolescent (13–18 years)
1. **B**edtime problems	Does your child have any problems going to bed? Falling asleep?	Does your child have any problems at bedtime? (P) Do you have any problems going to bed? (C)	Do you have any problems falling asleep at bedtime? (C)
2. **E**xcessive daytime sleepiness	Does your child seem overtired or sleepy a lot during the day? Does she still take naps?	Does your child have difficulty waking in the morning, seem sleepy during the day or take naps? (P) Do you feel tired a lot? (C)	Do you feel sleepy a lot during the day? In school? While driving? (C)
3. **A**wakenings during the night	Does your child wake up a lot at night?	Does your child seem to wake up a lot at night? Any sleepwalking or nightmares? (P) Do you wake up a lot at night? Have trouble getting back to sleep? (C)	Do you wake up a lot at night? Have trouble getting back to sleep? (C)
4. **R**egularity and duration of sleep	Does your child have a regular bedtime and wake time? What are they?	What time does your child go to bed and get up on school days? Weekends? Do you think he/she is getting enough sleep? (P)	What time do you usually go to bed on school nights? Weekends? How much sleep do you usually get? (C)
5. **S**noring	Does your child snore a lot or have difficulty breathing at night?	Does your child have loud or nightly snoring or any breathing difficulties at night? (P)	Does your teenager snore loudly or nightly? (P)

(P) Parent-directed question
(C) Child-directed question.

2

Biology of Sleep

Sleep organization and the regulation of sleep and wakefulness are complex, highly active physiologic processes that involve the interaction of multiple central nervous system components and impact on many other organ systems in the body (e.g., cardiovascular, respiratory, endocrine). A detailed description of the neuroanatomy and neurophysiology of sleep, which may be found in a number of excellent reviews (see "Suggested References"), is beyond the scope of this book. However, some understanding of the basic structure or architecture of sleep and familiarity with the basic mechanisms that regulate sleep and wakefulness are necessary in order to fully appreciate normal development (ontogeny) of sleep, as well as the causes and effects of sleep disturbances and inadequate sleep in children and adolescents.

While We Sleep

Sleep, although in some ways the "opposite" of wakefulness, is hardly an inert state. It shares many features with the alert state and is an active process during which many physiologic, metabolic, and neurobehavioral functions are ongoing and are organized within highly complex relationships.

FUNCTION OF SLEEP

Despite the explosion of knowledge in the past half-century regarding the structure, neuroanatomy, and neurophysiology of sleep (the discovery of REM sleep occurred barely 50 years ago), the basic function of sleep largely remains a mystery. Most of what we understand about the function of sleep has evolved from studies that have examined the impact of experimentally induced sleep loss or pathologic sleep conditions on a host of physiologic and neurobehavioral systems in both animal models and humans. We do know that adequate sleep is a biological imperative that appears necessary for sustaining life, as well as for optimal functioning; and clearly "rest" is not a substitute for sleep. For example, REM sleep appears not only to be involved in vital cognitive functions, such as the consolidation of memory, but to be an integral component of the growth and development of the central nervous system. In addition, the release of growth hormone during slow-wave sleep clearly links sleep to the regulation of somatic growth, as well as to many other neuroendocrine functions. Sleep may also functionally reflect a neurobiological need to limit time in the awake state, thereby protecting the individual, especially the developing organism, from being bombarded by information and environmental stimulation that cannot be adequately processed.

SLEEP ARCHITECTURE

The framework or architecture of sleep is based on recognition of two distinct sleep stages: *REM sleep* (rapid eye movement or "dream" sleep) and *non-REM sleep*. These stages are defined by distinct polysomnographic (or "overnight sleep study") features of electroencephalographic (EEG) patterns, eye movement, and muscle tone.

- **Non-REM sleep** may be viewed as a period of relatively low brain activity during which the regulatory capacity of the brain is actively ongoing and in which body movements are preserved. Non-REM sleep is further divided as follows:
  - **Stage 1** sleep occurs at the sleep–wake transition and is often referred to as "light sleep." Initial stage 1 typically lasts from 30 seconds to 5 minutes. Recall of fragmented visual imagery or hypnogogic hallucinations may occur, as may brief involuntary muscle contractions (hypnic jerks), both normal phenomena in most cases.
  - **Stage 2** sleep is usually considered the initiation of "true" sleep. It is characterized by bursts of rhythmic rapid EEG activity called sleep spindles (fluctuating episodes of fast activity) and high-amplitude slow-wave spikes called K complexes. The initial stage 2 period lasts from 5 to 25 minutes (Fig. 2.1).
  - **Stages 3 and 4** are otherwise known as "deep" sleep, slow-wave sleep, or delta sleep. This stage of sleep is characterized by delta waves. (Stage 3 is scored on a polysomnogram when delta waves occupy between 20% and 50% of the EEG activity, and stage 4 when delta accounts for more than 50%). Respiration is slowest and most regular during slow-wave sleep. The highest arousal threshold (most difficult to awaken) also occurs during slow-wave sleep; the lowest arousal threshold (easiest to awaken) is in stage 1. The initial slow-wave sleep period is about 30 to 45 minutes and is followed by a brief arousal (change to a lighter sleep stage) (Fig. 2.2).
- **REM sleep** is characterized by paralysis or nearly absent muscle tone (except for control of breathing and erectile tissue), high levels of cortical activity (low voltage, mixed frequency) that are associated with dreaming, and episodic bursts of phasic eye movements that are the hallmark of REM sleep. Irregular respiration and heart rate are also features. The first REM sleep period occurs about 70 to 100 minutes after sleep onset (REM onset latency) and lasts about 5 minutes (Fig. 2.3).

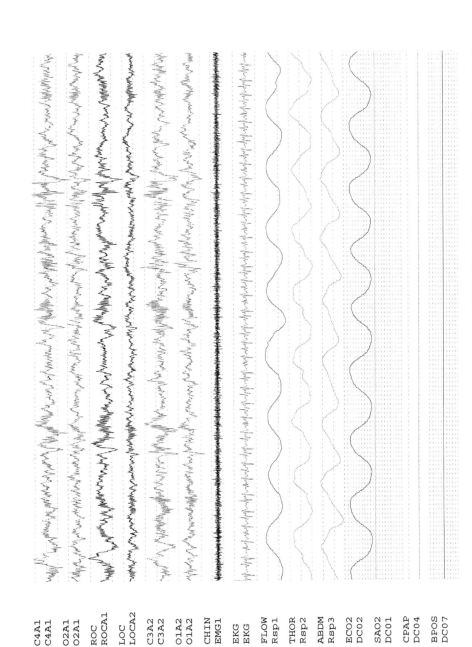

FIG. 2.1. Normal stage 2 sleep. Note sleep spindles and K-complexes in C4A1.

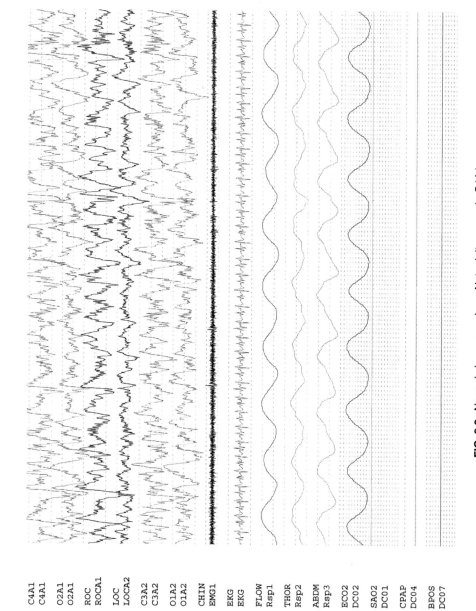

C4A1
C4A1
O2A1
O2A1
ROC
ROCA1
LOC
LOCA2
C3A2
C3A2
O1A2
O1A2
CHIN
EMG1
EKG
EKG
FLOW
Rsp1
THOR
Rsp2
ABDM
Rsp3
ECO2
DC02
SAO2
DC01
CPAP
DC04
BPOS
DC07

FIG. 2.2. Normal slow-wave sleep. Note delta waves in C4A1.

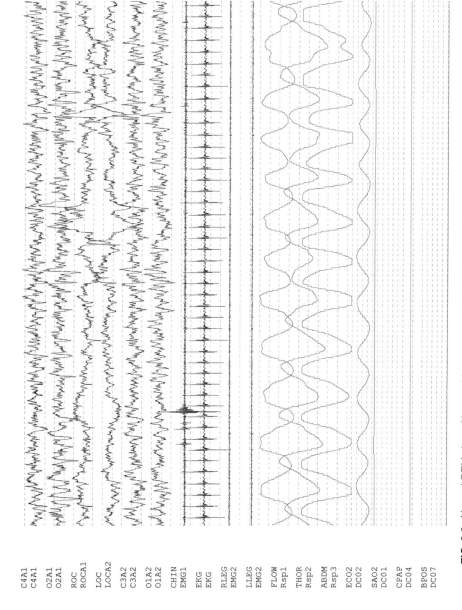

FIG. 2.3. Normal REM sleep. Note rapid eye movements in ROC and LOC, as well as irregular respiration in FLOW, THOR, and ABDM.

15

Sleep Stage Percentages in Healthy Young Adults	
Non-REM (total)	75%–80%
• Stage 1	2%–5%
• Stage 2	45%–55%
• Stage 3/4	3%–23%
REM	20%–25%, 4–6 episodes/night

Sleep cycles. Non-REM and REM sleep alternate throughout the night in cycles (*ultradian* cycles or rhythm) of about 90 to 110 minutes (50 minutes in infancy and gradually lengthening through childhood to adult levels). Brief arousals normally followed by a rapid return to sleep often occur at the end of each sleep cycle (four to six times per night). The relative proportion of REM and non-REM sleep per cycle changes across the night such that slow-wave sleep predominates in the first third of the night and REM sleep in the last third. That is, REM sleep percentage increases and slow-wave sleep percentage declines over the course of the night.

The amount and timing of each sleep stage are affected by a multitude of factors. For example, slow-wave sleep is linked to sleep onset and the length of prior wakefulness, whereas REM sleep is primarily linked to circadian body temperature rhythms. The relative percentage of sleep stages on a given night is also a reflection of other factors such as prior sleep loss (leads to increased percentage of slow-wave sleep during subsequent "recovery" sleep), circadian rhythm disruption associated with shift work or jet lag (causes disruption of timing of REM sleep), and medications, which have both direct effects and withdrawal effects, especially on slow-wave sleep and REM sleep (see Chapter 19).

ONTOGENY OF SLEEP

Sleep also changes as a function of age. Figure 2.4 illustrates the normal distribution of sleep stages in healthy children, adults, and the elderly. Both the emergence of these defined stages and the proportion of sleep that each occupies have a distinct ontogenic/developmental pattern (summarized in Table 2.1). As children mature, they assume more adult sleep patterns (shorter sleep duration, longer sleep cycles, less daytime sleep; see Chapter 3 for a more detailed discussion of the development of sleep patterns and behaviors across infancy and childhood). In particular, there is a dramatic decrease in the proportion of REM sleep from birth (50% of sleep) through early childhood into adulthood (25% to 30%), and an initial predominance of slow-wave sleep that peaks in early childhood, drops off abruptly after puberty, and then declines over the life span. Although the developmental significance of the preponderance of REM sleep in early life remains an area of active investigation, accumulated empirical evidence supports the hypothesis that the activation of autonomic and central nervous system processes in REM sleep helps to stimulate neuronal development.

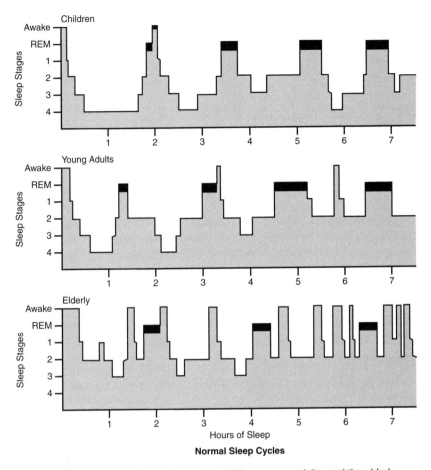

FIG. 2.4. Histogram of normal sleep for children, young adults, and the elderly.

Sleep Architecture and Clinical Sleep Disorders

A basic knowledge of sleep architecture and its developmental changes is also useful in understanding the underlying etiology of many sleep disorders. For example, the nightwakings commonly experienced by infants and toddlers are most often prolongations of the normal nighttime arousals that occur at the end of each (ultradian) sleep cycle. The partial arousal parasomnias (sleepwalking and sleep terrors) usually occur within 1 to 2 hours following sleep onset because that is when slow-wave sleep is predominant. In addition, the high prevalence of sleepwalking and sleep terrors in preschool-aged children is related to the relative increased proportion of slow-wave sleep in this age group. Finally, factors that increase the relative percentage of slow-wave sleep (withdrawal of slow-wave sleep suppressant medication, sleep deprivation) increase the likelihood of having a partial arousal episode.

TABLE 2.1. *Normal developmental changes in children's sleep architecture*

Age category	Average sleep duration (24 hr)	Sleep patterns	Sleep physiology
Newborns	16–20 hr	• 1- to 4-hr sleep periods followed by 1- to 2-hr awake periods • Amount daytime sleep = amount nighttime sleep	• 3 sleep states: active ("REM-like"; 50% of sleep), quiet ("non-REM-like"), and indeterminate • Enter sleep through active state
Infants (0–1 yr)	14–15 hr total at 4 mo; 13–14 hr total at 6 mo	• Sleep periods 3–4 hr first 3 mo; 6- to 8-hr periods at 4–6 mo • Day/night differentiation develops between 6 wk and 3 mo • 70%–80% "settle" (sleep through the night) at 9 mo • Naps: 2–4 hr in 2 naps/d	• Amount of active/REM sleep declines • Development of 4 stages of non-REM sleep • Sleep cycles every 50 min • Enter sleep through non-REM
Toddlers (1–3 yr)	12 hr total	• Nap 1.5–3.5 hr (1 nap/d)	• REM sleep amounts continue to decline
Preschool (3–6 yr)	11–12 hr	• Napping declines; most stop by age 5 yr	• REM sleep amounts continue to decline • Sleep cycles every 90 min • High levels of slow-wave sleep
Middle childhood (6–12 yr)	10–11 hr	• Low levels of daytime sleepiness • Increased discrepancy between school/nonschool night sleep amounts	• Latency from sleep onset to REM sleep increases • High sleep efficiency (time asleep/time in bed)
Adolescence (>12 yr)	9 hr ideal; 7 hr actual	• Often irregular sleep schedule • Circadian phase delay postpuberty with later bedtimes/earlier rise times	• 40% decline in slow-wave sleep • REM sleep at adult levels (25%–30%)

REM, rapid eye movement.

NEUROANATOMY/PHYSIOLOGY OF SLEEP

From a neuroanatomic standpoint, the key areas of the brain involved in the production and regulation of sleep are the brainstem, diencephalon, thalamus, and cerebral cortex. The "opposing" process of wakefulness is actively promoted by groups of cells in the reticular formation of the brainstem, which then activate the cortex. Neurotransmitters, hormones, and a number of neuropeptides actively modulate and influence these neuroanatomic substrates. These complex relationships help to explain the powerful sleep effects of drugs that alter the metabolism of these systems. For instance, sleep-promoting benzodiazepines enhance γ-aminobutyric acid (GABA) and wakefulness-promoting caffeine blocks adenosine receptors (see Chapter 19). Dopaminergic, monoaminergic, histaminergic, and cholinergic systems help sustain wakefulness, most likely mediated through the recently discovered "narcolepsy" peptide hypocretin (orexin). Serotonergic and GABAminergic neurons, adenosine (non-REM sleep), and cholinergics (REM sleep), as well as naturally occurring opiates, all have important roles in the sleep regulation.

SLEEP REGULATION

Sleep and wakefulness are regulated by two basic highly coupled processes operating simultaneously (the "two process" sleep system):

- **Homeostatic process,** which primarily regulates the length and depth of sleep.
- **Endogenous circadian rhythms** ("biological time clocks"), which influence the internal organization of sleep and timing and duration of daily sleep–wake cycles.

The relative level of sleepiness (sleep propensity) or alertness existing at any given time during a 24-hour period is partially determined by the duration and quality of previous sleep, as well as time awake since the last sleep period. Interacting with this "sleep homeostat" is a 24-hour cyclic pattern or rhythm characterized by clock-dependent periods of maximum sleepiness (*"circadian troughs"*) and maximum alertness (*"circadian nadirs"*). There are two periods of maximum sleepiness, one in the late afternoon and one in the middle of the night, and two periods of maximum alertness, one in the early morning and one in the evening. In addition, relative sleepiness and wakefulness are influenced by many other variables, including individual factors (e.g., age, individual variations in sleep needs and tolerance to the effects of inadequate sleep); the nature of the task being performed (e.g., type, length, complexity); and environmental factors (e.g., noise, ambient temperature) that may "unmask" *but do not cause* sleepiness.

Finally, a phenomenon known as *sleep inertia,* defined as a period of incomplete arousal characterized by confusion, impaired judgment, and poor memory consolidation occurring immediately upon waking from sleep, may further compromise alertness levels (particularly in the early morning) (Fig. 2.5).

In addition to having an inherent periodicity, intrinsic circadian rhythms are synchronized or "entrained" to the 24-hour-day cycle by environmental cues called *"zeitgebers."* In the absence of zeitgebers (what is termed the "free-running state"), circadian rhythms are desynchronized or "uncoupled" from one another. The most powerful of these zeitgebers is the light–dark cycle; light signals are transmitted to the suprachiasmatic nucleus (SCN) via the circadian photoreceptor system within the retina (functionally and anatomically separate from the visual system), which switch the body's production of the hormone *mela-*

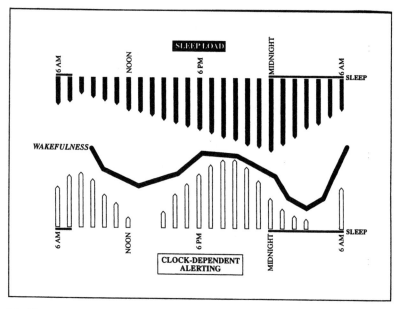

FIG. 2.5. Normal distribution of sleep stages in healthy children, adults, and the elderly. (From Dement WC, Vaughan C. *The promise of sleep: a pioneer in sleep medicine explores the vital connection between health, happiness, and a good night's sleep.* New York: Delacorte Press, 1999.)

tonin off (light) or on (dark). Circadian rhythms are also synchronized by other external time cues, such as timing of meals and alarm clocks. Thus, daytime schedules that are not consistently regulated may result in sleep disturbances. Finally, recent research also supports an important role for genetics in determining intrinsic circadian clock periodicities and, thus, influencing individual circadian preference for sleep–wake cycle timing ("night owl" versus "morning lark").

SLEEP LOSS

A basic principle of sleep physiology relates to the consequences of the failure to meet basic sleep needs. Most of the studies that have examined the effects of inadequate sleep on human beings have used conditions of total sleep loss (*sleep deprivation*) rather than the more "real world" scenario of partial sleep loss (*sleep restriction*). However, more recent studies have demonstrated that partial sleep loss on a chronic basis accumulates in what is termed a *sleep debt* that produces deficits equivalent to those seen under conditions of total sleep deprivation. If the sleep debt becomes large enough and is not voluntarily paid back (by obtaining adequate *recovery sleep*), the body may respond by overriding voluntary control of wakefulness, resulting in periods of decreased alertness, dozing off, and napping. In addition, the sleep-deprived individual may experience very brief (several seconds) repeated daytime *microsleeps* of which he or she may be completely unaware, but which nonetheless may result in significant lapses in attention and vigilance. There also appears to be a relationship between the amount of sleep restriction and performance, with decreased performance correlating with decreased sleep. Furthermore, subjective perception of sleepiness and the degree of associated performance impairment tend to be poorly correlated with actual impairment, frequently leading individuals to overestimate their ability to function with sleep loss.

Individual Sleep Needs

Individual sleep needs are dependent on a number of factors, including age. Recent research also indicates that tolerance for inadequate sleep appears to vary across individuals. That is, some individuals appear to function better or worse following sleep deprivation than others. Although the general profile of performance deficits following sleep loss is fairly consistent in human beings (e.g., compromise of efficiency, deterioration of performance over time), there may also be individual variation in relative susceptibility to the effects of inadequate sleep across domains (e.g., memory, attention, mood).

3

Sleep in Infancy, Childhood, and Adolescence

GENERAL CONSIDERATIONS

The evaluation of pediatric sleep problems first and foremost requires a basic understanding of what constitutes "normal" sleep in infants, children, and adolescents. Sleep disturbances, as well as many characteristics of sleep itself, have some distinctly different features in children from those in adults. In addition, normal sleep architecture, sleep patterns, and sleep behaviors evolve and change significantly as children progress from infancy to middle childhood through adolescence.

Furthermore, appreciation and understanding of these changes are also needed to provide parents with anticipatory guidance regarding normal sleep and sleep patterns at different developmental stages. For example, an important component of sleep physiology that is particularly relevant to understanding sleep in children is the ontogeny of sleep consolidation and regulation. *Consolidation* of the nocturnal sleep period ("sleeping through the night") requires the ability to sustain increasingly longer sleep periods and to shift to primarily nighttime sleep. Because this developmental progression occurs over the first few months of life, parents should be counseled not to expect their infant to sleep through the night until about 3 months of age. *Sleep regulation* involves the ability to control internal states of arousal more effectively as an infant matures, which eventually enables the infant to fall asleep at bedtime and to fall back asleep during the night on his or her own. Thus, anticipatory guidance counseling to put a baby to sleep "drowsy but awake" is most appropriately initiated at the 2-month visit, so that parents can begin to develop good sleep habits as their baby begins to develop the ability to self-soothe.

The relative prevalence and the various types of sleep problems that occur throughout childhood must also be understood in the context of normal physical and cognitive/emotional phenomena that are occurring at different developmental stages. For example, normal separation anxiety in toddlers may be associated with increased nighttime fears and problematic nightwakings, and the prevalence of obstructive sleep apnea in preschoolers is linked to the relative prominence of lymphoid tissue (adenotonsillar hypertrophy) in early childhood. Parental identification and reporting of sleep problems in children also varies across childhood, with parents of infants and toddlers more likely to be aware of sleep concerns than those of school-aged children and adolescents. The very definition of a "sleep problem" by parents is often highly subjective and is frequently determined by the amount of disruption caused to parents' sleep.

In addition to considering sleep disturbances in a developmental context, it is important for the clinician to recognize that a number of other important child, parental, and environmental variables affect the type, relative prevalence, chronicity, and severity of sleep problems. Child variables that may significantly impact sleep include temperament and behavioral style, individual variations in circadian preference, medical problems, delays in development, and acute and chronic stress. Parental variables include parenting styles, parents' educational level and knowledge of child development, mental health issues, family stress, and quality and quantity of parents' sleep and fatigue level. Environmental variables include the physical environment (space, sleeping arrangements); family composition (number, ages, and health status of siblings and extended family members); lifestyle issues (working parents, regularity of daily schedule); and cultural issues and family values (importance and meaning of sleep, acceptance of co-sleeping).

Nature vs. Nurture

Sleep habits, in general, may be viewed as *learned behaviors* superimposed on fundamental processes of circadian and sleep biology that, in turn, may be modified by genetic factors and developmental changes.

A description of normal sleep patterns, developmental issues, common parental sleep concerns, prevalence and types of common sleep problems, and other sleep issues in different age groups is provided below. Suggested specific anticipatory guidance points to emphasize during well-child visits are listed at the end of the chapter.

What Is "Enough" Sleep?

The simple answer to the question is "the amount of sleep that a child needs to feel well rested." Parents are generally quite good at recognizing the signs that indicate that their child is "overtired" (whininess, moodiness, short fuse, acting "hyper") at the end of the day, but may need help in recognizing that more subtle variations of these signs may be evidence of chronically inadequate sleep.

The numbers given below for average sleep duration at different ages represent the best information that is currently available. Recent research in adults and some preliminary data in children suggest, however, that there are individual variations in both sleep needs and tolerance levels to inadequate sleep, within certain basic parameters of human sleep needs. If parents are uncertain as to the amount of sleep their child needs to *function optimally*, monitoring sleep amounts and mood while allowing a child to sleep until he or she awakens spontaneously in the morning for at least 3 days (during vacation, for example) may help in sorting out this issue.

NEWBORNS (0 TO 2 MONTHS)

Normal Sleeping Patterns

- **Hours of sleep.** 16 to 20 hours per 24 hours, may be higher in premature babies; bottle-fed babies generally sleep for longer periods (3 to 5 hour) than breast-fed babies (2 to 3 hours asleep); sleep periods are separated by 1 to 3 hours awake.
- No nocturnal/diurnal pattern in first few weeks; sleep is distributed throughout the day and night.

Developmental Issues That May Impact Sleep

- Sleep–wake cycles are largely dependent on hunger and satiety; circadian rhythms and environmental cues play a much smaller role in newborns than with older infants.

Common Sleep Issues

- **Day/night reversal:** Day/night reversal is common in the first few weeks; increasing the infant's activity during the day and promoting dim lights at night will help align sleep with nighttime.
- **Irregular sleep patterns:** Regular rhythm of periods of sleepiness and alertness will emerge by 2 to 4 months.

- **Active vs. quiet sleep:** The smiling, grimacing, sucking, snuffling, and body movements such as twitches and jerks that are typical of active sleep in infants may be misinterpreted by parents as "restless" or disturbed sleep.
- **Sleeping environment:** Options include a bassinet/crib in sibling or baby's own room or bassinet/crib in parent's room. Sleeping in the parental bed may pose a risk of accidental suffocation. The infant's bedroom and surrounding environment (e.g., lighting) should be the same at bedtime as it will be throughout the night.
- **Sleeping surface:** Safety and prevention of suffocation are key considerations. Crib mattresses should provide a firm sleeping surface, fit tightly in the crib, and no pillows or comforters should be used. The distance between crib slats should be no greater than 2-⅜ inches.
- **Sleeping position:** Empirical studies have clearly demonstrated that sleeping on the back or in the side position reduces the risk of sudden infant death syndrome (SIDS).

Safe Sleep Practices for Infants

- Place the baby on his or her back to sleep at night and during naptime.
- Place the baby on a firm mattress in a safety-approved crib.
- Make sure the baby's face and head stay uncovered and clear of blankets and other coverings during sleep. If a blanket is used, make sure the baby is placed "feet to foot" (feet at the bottom of the crib, blanket no higher than chest level, blanket tucked in around mattress) in the crib.
- Create a "smoke-free zone" around the baby.
- Avoid overheating during sleep and maintain the baby's bedroom at a temperature comfortable for an average adult.
- Remove all mobiles and hanging crib toys by about 5 months, when the baby begins to pull up in the crib.
- Remove crib bumpers by about 12 months, when the baby can begin to climb.

- **Parental sleep:** Parental sleep also needs to be a priority; sleep deprivation is associated with maternal mood changes and may be a risk factor for maternal postpartum depression.

Prevalence of Sleep Problems

Most sleep issues that are perceived as problematic at this stage represent a discrepancy between parental expectations and developmentally appropriate sleep behaviors. Infants who are noted by parents to be extremely fussy and persistently difficult to console are more likely to have underlying medical issues, such as colic, gastroesophageal reflux, and formula intolerance.

Other Important Concepts

• Parents should be encouraged to learn to recognize both their newborn's intrinsic sleep–wake rhythms and signs of drowsiness (e.g., eye rubbing, irritability, yawning); delaying the opportunity to sleep when these signs occur may result in more difficulty settling.

INFANTS (2 TO 12 MONTHS)

Normal Sleeping Patterns

• **Hours of sleep:** Nighttime: 9 to 12 hours; naps: 2 to 4.5 hours.
• **Naps:** 4 to 1; with fewer as they get older; each lasting from 30 minutes to 2 hours.

Developmental Issues That May Impact Sleep

• Issues of attachment and social interaction are felt to play an important role in shaping sleep behaviors. For example, infants who are insecurely attached have been reported to have more sleep problems, although sleep problems do not necessarily imply attachment concerns. On the other hand, studies have shown that infants who are more socially engaged with their caretaker may be more reluctant to interrupt social interactions at bedtime for sleep!

Sleep as a Social Behavior

Sleep behavior in infancy, in particular, must be understood in the context of the *relationship* and *interaction* between child and caregiver, which impacts greatly on the quality and quantity of sleep.

• Acquisition of gross motor developmental milestones (e.g., rolling over, pulling to standing) and other such events may temporarily disrupt sleep; increased mobility increases the likelihood of limit-setting issues at bedtime.
• As object permanence develops in the second half of the first year, separation anxiety may result in increased bedtime resistance and problematic nightwakings.

Common Sleep Issues

- **Sleep regulation** or "self-soothing" involves the infant's ability to negotiate the sleep–wake transition both at sleep onset and following normal awakenings throughout the night.
- **Sleep consolidation** or "sleeping through the night," although often operationally defined by researchers as a period of sleep without waking from midnight to 5 AM, is usually defined by parents as a continuous sleep episode without the need for parental intervention (e.g., feeding, soothing) from the child's bedtime through the early morning. Studies suggest that about 70% to 80% of infants sleep through the night by 9 months.
- **Sleep onset associations** are those conditions that are present at the time that the infant falls asleep and may include being rocked, held, bottle fed, and breast fed. These conditions may be required again following normal nighttime arousals.
- **Nighttime arousals** are a consequence of the normal ultradian rhythm of 90- to 120-minute sleep cycles. All infants and children normally arouse briefly on average 4 to 6 times throughout the night. Characterization of these nighttime arousals include the following considerations:
  - **"Self-soothers" vs. "non-self-soothers":** Babies who soothe themselves back to sleep generally experience brief arousals rather than prolonged nightwakings. This capacity to self-soothe is associated with the practice of being put to bed while drowsy but still awake and without sleep onset associations that will be unavailable during the night. It may be beneficial to suggest to parents that they help their infant develop appropriate sleep onset associations that will be readily available to the infant during the night without the need for parental intervention (e.g., falling asleep independently in crib, thumbsucking, use of a transitional object).
  - **"Signalers" vs. "nonsignalers":** During nighttime arousals/wakings, infants may alert (signal) parents by crying or may return to sleep without disrupting parental sleep (nonsignalers). Not surprisingly, signalers are more likely to be labeled by parents as having problematic sleep. It has been estimated that 20% to 30% of 1-year-olds are considered to be signalers.
  - **Parental intervention vs. nonintervention:** Parents choose whether or not to respond to a signaled or nonsignaled arousal/awakening by such behaviors as verbal soothing, rocking, or feeding. The practice of parents responding immediately to signaled nightwakings, particularly if the interaction is reinforcing for the infant, may result in a "trained night crier."
  - **Night-to-night variability:** It should be noted that there is often considerable night-to-night and week-to-week variability in all of these behaviors, and neither infants nor parents are always consistent in the way they behave and interact. However, it is clear that a pattern of persistent difficulty in self-soothing is associated with frequent and problematic nightwakings in infants.

- **Transitional objects,** such as a pacifier or a blanket, become important during infancy. Providing the same object at naptime may strengthen attachment to a transitional object. A television set is not a transitional object and should not be in the room where the baby sleeps or play a role in the regular bedtime routine. Some infants respond positively to the use of a mother's well-worn, knotted T-shirt (with her scent) as a comfort object.
- **Night feedings** have not been shown to increase the quality or quantity of sleep and, in most cases, are not physiologically necessary after 6 months of age.
  - If the bedtime transition to sleep onset routinely occurs in the context of bottle feeding (or nursing), night feeding may become a necessary component of the infant's returning to sleep following nightwakings. The need for feedings during the night may also become a learned behavior ("learned hunger"), which leads to more frequent and prolonged nightwakings. Frequent night feedings may also disrupt sleep by resulting in bladder distention and discomfort from soaked diapers. Finally, being put down to sleep with a nighttime bottle increases the risk of dental caries and otitis media.
  - Breast-fed babies are likely to awaken more frequently for feedings than bottle-fed babies.
  - Parents should be encouraged to wean the infant from middle-of-the-night feedings by 6 months and to avoid putting him or her to sleep with a bottle.

Prevalence of Sleep Problems

Many sleep "problems" that occur before the age of 6 months are defined as such because of a perceived maturational lag in meeting developmental sleep milestones (e.g., "sleeping through the night," settling at bedtime); thus, these "problems" are likely to be transient in nature. Others are the result of a mismatch between infant behavior and parental expectation. Temporary sleep disturbances that occur in conjunction with developmental milestones, as well as acute illnesses, also tend to be self-limited if parental behaviors that reinforce difficulty settling or nightwakings are avoided. However, not all infant sleep problems are transient, and certain factors appear to be associated with an increased risk of chronicity. These include inability to self-soothe, difficult temperament, maternal depression, and insecure maternal–child attachment.

It is estimated that about 25% to 50% of 6- to 12-month-olds and 30% of 1-year-olds have problematic nightwakings, and about 50% have sleep onset or settling difficulties at 12 months.

Common Sleep Disorders

- Sleep onset association disorder/nightwakings (see Chapter 7)
- Rhythmic movement disorders (headbanging, bodyrocking, bodyrolling) (see Chapter 11)

Other Important Concepts

- Most infants benefit from a set sleep schedule with regular naptimes and bed-time that reflects the infant's natural preferences for sleep and waking patterns, as well as family lifestyle issues.
- At the 2-month visit, parents may be encouraged to start putting the infant to bed drowsy but awake within the next 4 to 8 weeks.
- A consistent and enjoyable bedtime routine leading up to sleep onset can be established from the age of 3 months. The bedtime routine may include any of the following: feeding, bath, story, music, massage, rocking.
- Parents should be encouraged to take the opportunity to nap when the infant is sleeping.
- It is important to discuss the possibility with parents that their previously "great" sleeper may develop transitory problems with nightwakings and bed-time resistance during times of stress or in association with achievement of developmental milestones. Avoidance of parental reinforcement (e.g., with attention, night feedings) often prevents a small, temporary sleep problem from becoming a large and chronic one.

To Co-sleep or Not to Co-sleep

Co-sleeping or bed sharing is a topic that has clearly generated a consid-erable amount of controversy and discussion among both general and devel-opmental/behavioral pediatricians. The issues that have been raised in defending or decrying the practice of co-sleeping are myriad, ranging from the effects on the health of the co-sleeping infant (the practice is cited as both protective against and increasing the risk for SIDS, implicated in suf-focation deaths, and correlated with longer-term breast feeding) to both pos-itive and negative psychosocial and developmental effects (individuation vs. intimacy, sexual attitudes, attachment) to sociologic and anthropologic con-siderations as viewed in a family context (cultural and ethnic values).

The decision to co-sleep is made by families for a variety of reasons, which are important to explore in addressing this issue in the health care setting. Parents should be encouraged to share their practices and feel-ings; all too often, parents are reluctant to be honest about the practice of co-sleeping for fear of disapproval from the medical profession. It may be more useful to consider the strengths and vulnerabilities of the individual child, parent, and parent–child dyad in assessing the potential risks of co-sleeping in a given situation rather than adopting a "one size fits all" approach. Counseling parents on this issue requires a sensitive, open, and nondogmatic approach, the goal of which is to more effec-tively guide parents in making informed choices that are in their family's best interest.

TODDLERS (12 MONTHS TO 3 YEARS)

Normal Sleep Patterns

- **Hours of sleep:** 12 to 13 over 24 hours.
- **Naps** decrease from two naps to one at average age of 18 months.

Developmental Issues That May Impact Sleep

Gross motor: Independent locomotion results in increased ability to get out of bed and come into the parents' room during nightwakings.

Cognitive:
- Drive to learn, rapid acquisition of skills may result in difficulty settling at bedtime.
- Comprehension of cause and effect enables the child to respond to simple behavioral interventions.
- Understanding of the symbolic meaning of objects leads to increased interest in and reliance on transitional objects.
- Development of imagination and fantasy may result in increased nighttime fears.

Language:
- Expressive language development lags behind receptive, which may limit verbal expression of nighttime fears and concerns.

Social/emotional:
- The drive for autonomy and independence may lead to increased bedtime resistance.
- Separation anxiety peaks at 18 to 24 months and is often associated with increased nightwakings.
- Regression in behavior is a common stress response and may increase the likelihood of co-sleeping.

Common Sleep Issues

- **Naps.** There are many components that can raise concerns with naps, including number, duration, timing, location, giving up, and need for naps. Restricting naps will not help a child sleep better at night; however, placement of naps too close to the scheduled bedtime may interfere with sleep onset.
- **Transition from crib to bed.** This step is usually taken between 2 and 3 years of age, or when safety concerns related to falling while climbing out of the crib become an issue (although a mesh crib tent can alleviate safety concerns). The transition to a bed at too young an age can result in the development of sleep problems.
- **Bedtime bottles and night feedings.** As noted in the section on infants, the bedtime transition to sleep onset ideally occurs without a feeding in order to

facilitate independent settling. The same issues as described in infants in terms of learned hunger, arousals related to bladder distention, dental caries, and increased risk of otitis media associated with nighttime bottles apply to toddlers as well.

- **Bedtime routines** are an important daily ritual for parents to develop and maintain in order to help ease the transition from high levels of activity during the day to sleep onset. The events of the bedtime routine should be consistent, occur in the same temporal order, and be of an increasingly relaxing nature for that particular child as bedtime is neared.
- **Transitional objects** at bedtime and naptime, such as blankets, dolls, and stuffed animals, become increasingly important at this stage and help to foster independent settling and self-soothing. Thumbsucking and pacifiers before age 4 years, especially if limited to bedtime, is unlikely to result in significant orthodontic problems. Thumbsucking and pacifiers at this age should not be discouraged.

Prevalence of Sleep Problems

Sleep problems in toddlers are very common, occurring in 25% to 30% of this age group. Bedtime resistance found in 10% to 15% of toddlers, and nightwakings in 15% to 20%, are the two most common concerns of parents, followed by nighttime fears and nightmares. Sleep problems may also be persistent, especially in children with daytime behavior problems. Conversely, daytime behavior problems are more common in poor sleepers (45%).

Common Sleep Disorders

- Sleep onset association disorder/nightwakings (see Chapter 7)
- Limit setting sleep disorder/bedtime resistance (see Chapter 6)
- Rhythmic movement disorders (headbanging, bodyrocking, bodyrolling) (see Chapter 11)

Other Important Concepts

- Secondary prevention involves avoiding reinforcement of transitory sleep problems and preventing a sleep disturbance from becoming a sleep disorder.
- Sleep disturbances are often manifested in daytime behavior as a result of the bidirectional effects of sleep on behavior.
- It should be noted that in children with nightwaking problems, there may be a "golden" window of opportunity to initiate a graduated extinction program before the child is transitioned to a bed and is, thus, able to come into the parents' bedroom during the night.

PRESCHOOL-AGED CHILDREN (3 TO 5 YEARS)

Normal Sleep Patterns

- **Hours of sleep:** 11 to 12 over 24 hours
- **Naps** decrease from one nap to no nap.

Developmental Issues That May Impact Sleep

- Expanded language and cognitive skills may lead to increased bedtime resistance, as children become more articulate about their needs and may engage in more limit-testing behavior.
- A developing capacity to delay gratification and anticipate consequences enables preschoolers to respond to positive reinforcement for appropriate bedtime behavior.
- Further development of imagination and fantasy may heighten nighttime fears.
- Increasing interest in developing literacy skills reinforces the importance of reading aloud at bedtime as an integral part of the bedtime routine.

Common Sleep Issues

- **Naps:** A large percentage of children stop napping between the ages of 3 and 4, with many children continuing to nap up to age 5 (Table 3.1).
- **Co-sleeping:** Persistent co-sleeping tends to be highly associated with sleep problems in this age group.
- **Sleep schedules:** Preschoolers need a set, consistent bedtime and waketime. A regular and consistent daytime routine (e.g., meals, playtimes) also helps to regularize the sleep–wake schedule. Children who are not in morning school or day care settings may do fine with a relatively later bedtime but may need to readjust their schedule once school starts. Parents should be encouraged to start this gradual process several weeks in advance of the anticipated change in morning schedule.
- **Second wind or "forbidden zone":** This often reflects the late-day circadian-mediated surge in alertness that occurs in everyone, but may have an exaggerated behavioral component in some children. If (attempted) bedtime coincides

TABLE 3.1. *Napping statistics in young children*

Age (yr)	% Still napping
3	92
4	57
5	27

with this circadian peak, the likely result is bedtime resistance. Delaying the bedtime, or moving the bedtime earlier, when the child is more physiologically ready for sleep, often successfully addresses the problem of a child being consistently wide awake at bedtime.

Prevalence of Sleep Problems

Difficulties falling asleep and nightwakings (15% to 30%) are still common in this age group, in many cases coexisting in the same child (average time to fall asleep in this age group is around 15 minutes). A number of studies have suggested that sleep problems in this age group may become chronic; in one study, 84% of children aged 15 to 48 months with bedtime struggles and/or nightwaking continued to have significant sleep disturbance at 3-year follow-up.

Common Sleep Disorders

- Nighttime fears and nightmares (see Chapters 8 and 9)
- Sleep onset association disorder/nightwakings (see Chapter 7)
- Limit-setting sleep disorder/bedtime resistance (see Chapter 6)
- Obstructive sleep apnea and sleep disordered breathing (see Chapter 13)
- Partial arousal parasomnias (sleepwalking, sleep terrors) (see Chapter 10)

Other Important Concepts

- The association between inadequate or disturbed sleep and behavioral problems tends to become more evident at this age.
- Parents should be encouraged to make reading an integral part of the bedtime routine.

SCHOOL-AGED CHILDREN (6 TO 12 YEARS)

Normal Sleeping Patterns

Hours of sleep: 10 to 11 hours over 24 hours

Wake-up Call

Napping and persistent complaints or behavioral manifestation of daytime sleepiness reported by parents or teachers in school-aged children are a red flag. These suggest significant problems with sleep quality and/or quantity or, less frequently, a primary disorder of excessive daytime sleepiness. Such complaints should be taken seriously and evaluated carefully by the primary care provider.

Developmental Issues That May Impact Sleep

Cognitive:
- Comprehension of existence of real dangers (e.g., burglars) may increase nighttime fears.

Social/emotional:
- Increasing independence from parental supervision and a shift in responsibility for health habits as children approach adolescence may result in less enforcement of appropriate bedtimes and inadequate sleep duration; parents may also be less aware of sleep problems if they do exist.

Healthy Sleep/Healthy Child

Middle childhood is a critical time for the development of health habits in general and healthy sleep habits in particular. Practitioners have a real opportunity in the context of well-child care to introduce concepts of sleep health promotion (good sleep habits) and disease prevention (impact of inadequate sleep) to children at this stage, and studies suggest that middle school–aged children may be particularly receptive to counseling and education about sleep from their primary care provider.

- Involvement in academic, social, athletic, and family activities, as well as parent work schedules, may conflict with time for sleep.
- Increasing reliance on peer relationships.
- Social anxiety and need for academic achievement may result in nighttime worrying, interfering with sleep onset.
- Media and electronics, such as television, computer, video games, and the internet, all compete increasingly for sleep time.

The Electronic Sandman

Television viewing at bedtime and the presence of a television set in the child's bedroom in particular have been found to be associated with difficulties in falling and staying asleep in children. Television may also play a role in increasing the likelihood of nightmares and nighttime anxiety. Parents should be encouraged to keep electronic media devices out of the sleeping environment.

Common Sleep Issues

- **Irregularity of sleep–wake schedules** reflects increasing discrepancy between school and nonschool night bedtimes and waketimes.
- **Increased caffeine intake** may interfere with sleep onset and quality of sleep.
- **Daytime sleepiness** is rare in this population, therefore, parents should be encouraged to report any persistent daytime sleepiness.

Prevalence of Sleep Problems

Although conventional wisdom has previously indicated that sleep problems are rare in middle childhood, recent studies have reported an overall prevalence of significant parent-reported sleep problems of 37% in this age group, with a 15% to 25% prevalence of bedtime resistance, a 10% prevalence of significant sleep onset delay and anxiety at bedtime, and a 10% prevalence of teacher- and parent-reported daytime sleepiness. It should also be noted that these figures might underestimate the magnitude of sleep problems because parents may be unaware of and, thus, underreport sleep concerns at this age.

Common Sleep Disorders

- Sleepwalking and sleep terrors (see Chapter 10)
- Bruxism (see Chapter 12)
- Obstructive sleep apnea and sleep disordered breathing (see Chapter 13)
- Insufficient sleep (see Chapter 18)
- Inadequate sleep hygiene (see Chapter 18)

Other Important Concepts

- **Maturational issues:** Many of the developmental sleep changes associated with puberty described in the following section on adolescent sleep may be applicable to the early-maturing middle school–aged child.
- **Circadian preference:** Recent data suggest that individuals may begin to manifest an inherent relative lifelong circadian sleep phase preference ("morningness–eveningness," "night owl vs. morning lark") in childhood. Children who are relatively phase delayed (e.g., prefer a later bedtime and rise time) may display sleep onset problems and associated bedtime resistance when given a bedtime that is significantly earlier than their preferred sleep onset time but fall asleep easily and quickly when given a later bedtime. Allowing a child to sleep on a *self-selected* sleep schedule for several days (e.g., during vacation) may help to clarify the issue of circadian preference.

Owls and Larks

Parents and providers should be sensitive to circadian preference, particularly for a delayed (later) sleep phase as a possible cause of bedtime struggles. Sleep schedules for these children may need to be adjusted accordingly to reduce sleep onset delay while preserving adequate sleep amounts.

- Encouragement of healthy sleep habits and an emphasis on the importance of adequate sleep by parents, teachers, and health care practitioners is particularly important in the middle childhood years and may set the stage for development of continued positive sleep behaviors in adolescence and adulthood.

ADOLESCENTS (12 TO 18 YEARS)

Normal Sleeping Patterns

Hours of sleep: 9 to 9½ hours needed on average; most teens get 7 to 7¼ hours.

Developmental Issues That May Impact Sleep

- Around the time of puberty onset, adolescents develop an approximately 2-hour physiologically based phase delay (later sleep onset and wake times), relative to sleep–wake cycles in middle childhood. This is a result of pubertal/hormonal influences on circadian sleep–wake cycles and melatonin secretion.
- Adolescent sleep needs do not differ dramatically from sleep needs of preadolescents, and optimal sleep amounts remain at about 9 to 9¼ hours per night. However, epidemiologic research on "normal" sleep patterns and amounts suggests that most adolescents obtain on the average of 7 to 7½ hours of sleep per night. This often results in the accumulation of a considerable sleep debt over time.
- Adolescents have a physiologic tendency to develop *decreased daytime alertness* levels in mid- to late puberty.

Common Sleep Issues

- Environmental factors and lifestyle/social demands, such as homework, after-school jobs, and social activities impact significantly on sleep cycles in adolescents, frequently resulting in delayed sleep onset.
- There is significant variability in sleep–wake patterns in adolescents from weekday to weekend.

- Early start times of many high schools, as well as middle and junior high schools, may result in premature waketimes in the morning and contribute to insufficient sleep.
- All of the above factors often combine to produce significant sleepiness in many adolescents and consequent impairment in mood, attention, memory, behavioral control, and academic performance. Parents of teenagers should be strongly encouraged to monitor their adolescent's sleep and possible negative consequences of sleep deprivation and to actively intervene if sleep is chronically inadequate.
- As with all adolescent risk-taking behavior, parents should be encouraged to maintain a level of open communication with their teenager regarding the impact of inadequate sleep and poor sleep habits on social/emotional functioning, school performance, and health.

Sleepy, Dopey, and Grumpy

There is now substantial evidence to suggest that adolescents in the United States, as a group, are chronically sleep deprived. Studies suggest that many teens function for a good part of the day in the "twilight zone," which is a level of sleepiness equivalent to that in individuals with narcolepsy! Practitioners should be aware of the potential for and carefully assess adolescent patients for chronic sleepiness, and the accompanying effects on mood, behavior, and school performance.

Prevalence of Sleep Problems

Data suggest that chronic partial sleep deprivation is a serious problem in this age group and that particular groups, including "high achievers" who are engaged in many extracurricular activities, may be at a relatively high risk. Chronic sleep restriction in adolescents can lead to significant neurobehavioral consequences, including a negative impact on mood, vigilance and reaction time, attention, memory, behavioral control, and motivation.

Adolescents may also suffer from a number of sleep disorders. A number of studies have suggested that the prevalence of significant sleep problems in adolescents is high (at least 20%) and that particular groups of adolescents, such as those with chronic medical or psychiatric problems (e.g., depression), may be at increased risk.

Common Sleep Disorders

- Insufficient sleep (see Chapter 18)
- Inadequate sleep hygiene (see Chapter 18)

- Insomnia (see Chapter 17)
- Delayed sleep phase syndrome (see Chapter 16)
- Restless legs syndrome/periodic limb movement disorder (see Chapter 14)
- Narcolepsy (see Chapter 15)

Other Important Concepts

Chronic insufficient sleep in adolescents may be associated with:

- Significant declines in school and work/occupational performance.
- Use of potentially harmful alertness-promoting agents such as caffeine and stimulant medications.
- Increased risk-taking behaviors (e.g., use of alcohol, illicit drugs), injuries, including occupational and sports injuries, and motor vehicle crashes.

Asleep at the Wheel

Older adolescent boys are among the highest risk groups for drowsy driving–related accidents. The most common drowsy driving accident involves a single vehicle with a single driver who drives off the road late at night. All adolescents with insufficient sleep are at risk, especially when lack of sleep is compounded by a beer or two, marijuana, and relative driving inexperience.

Practitioners should directly question adolescent patients about their sleep habits in order to obtain the most accurate and complete picture.

ANTICIPATORY GUIDANCE FOR SLEEP ISSUES IN INFANTS, CHILDREN, AND ADOLESCENTS

Prenatal Visit

- Discuss normal newborn sleep patterns (day/night reversal, sleep amounts per 24 hours, average sleep–wake periods).
- Discuss plans for sleeping arrangements.

Newborn Visit

- Discuss normal newborn sleep patterns (day/night reversal, sleep amounts per 24 hours, average sleep–wake periods, irregularity).
- Discuss specific safe sleep practices (sleeping position, surface, environment).
- Breast-fed baby: Discuss shorter sleep periods, avoidance of caffeine.
- Highlight importance of parental sleep needs.

2-Week Visit

- Review normal newborn sleep patterns (day/night reversal, normal range of total sleep per 24 hours, average sleep–wake periods, irregularity).
- Review safe sleep practices (sleeping position, surface, environment).
- Breast-fed baby: Discuss shorter sleep periods, avoidance of caffeine.
- Highlight importance of parental sleep needs.

2-Month Visit

- Discuss normal development of infant sleep patterns (normal range of total sleep per 24 hours, "sleeping through the night," self-soothing, appropriate sleep onset associations).
- Encourage parents to put their baby to sleep *drowsy but awake* starting at about 3 months of age to avoid the development of inappropriate sleep associations.
- Encourage parents to make the transition to final sleeping arrangements (e.g.., bassinet to crib; parents' room to baby's room) by 3 months.
- Explain to parents that periodic, brief arousals during the night are part of a baby's normal sleep pattern, which may help to avoid unnecessary parental intervention and subsequent reinforcement of nightwaking.
- Review safe sleep practices (sleeping position, surface, environment).
- Breast-fed baby: Discuss shorter sleep periods, avoidance of caffeine.
- Highlight importance of parental sleep needs.

4-Month Visit

- Discuss normal development of infant sleep patterns.
- Encourage parents to put their baby to sleep *drowsy but awake.*
- Discuss importance of a daily schedule with consistent meal times and sleep times.
- Suggest that during-the-night feedings should be discouraged after about 6 months, as they may contribute to inappropriate learned sleep behaviors and are no longer physiologically necessary for most healthy babies.
- Encourage establishment of a bedtime routine.
- Review safe sleep practices (sleeping position, surface, environment).

6-Month Visit

- Discuss normal development of infant sleep and napping patterns.
- Encourage parents to put their baby to sleep *drowsy but awake.*
- Suggest that during-the-night feedings should be discouraged after about 6 months, as they may contribute to inappropriate learned sleep behaviors and are no longer physiologically necessary for most healthy babies.
- Encourage establishment of a bedtime routine and consistent sleep schedule.
- Anticipate possible temporary regression in sleep behaviors with developmental milestones, illness, and changes in routine.
- Invite discussion of co-sleeping.

9-Month Visit

- Discuss normal development of infant sleep and napping patterns.
- Anticipate recurrence of nightwakings at 9 to 12 months; discourage parental reinforcement of nightwakings.
- Encourage establishment of a bedtime routine and consistent sleep schedule.
- Invite discussion of co-sleeping.

1-Year Visit

- Discuss normal development of toddler sleep and napping patterns.
- Discuss transition to single daily nap period.
- Encourage bedtime routine and regular bedtime.

15-Month Visit

- Discuss normal development of toddler sleep and napping patterns.
- Encourage use of transitional objects.
- Discuss transition to single daily nap period.
- Discourage bedtime bottles.

18-Month Visit

- Discuss normal development of toddler sleep and napping patterns.
- Encourage transitional objects.
- Discourage bedtime bottles.
- Discuss nighttime developmental fears (especially separation).
- Discourage television viewing at bedtime.

2-Year Visit

- Discuss normal development of toddler sleep and napping patterns.
- Discuss effects of inadequate sleep on daytime behavior.
- Discuss transition from crib to bed.
- Discuss parental limit setting.

3- to 5-Year Visits

- Discuss normal development of sleep and napping patterns in preschoolers.
- Discuss effects of inadequate sleep on daytime behavior and review signs of sleepiness.
- Discuss development of good sleep habits.
- Discuss parental limit setting.
- Discourage TV viewing at bedtime and suggest no TV set in the child's bedroom.

6- To 12-Year Visits

- Discuss normal range sleep amounts in school-aged children.
- Encourage obtaining adequate sleep and appropriate bedtime.
- Discuss impact of inadequate sleep on school performance.
- Discuss development of good sleep habits.
- Discourage TV at bedtime and suggest no TV set in the child's bedroom.

Adolescent Visits

- Discuss average sleep needs (9 to 9¼ hours) in teenagers.
- Encourage obtaining adequate sleep and appropriate bedtime.
- Discuss avoiding discrepant weekday and weekend schedules.
- Review pubertal influences on sleep (phase delay).
- Review healthy sleep habits (regular bedtimes and waketimes, avoidance of caffeine, avoidance of TV set/computers in bedroom).
- Discuss dangers of drowsy driving.

4

Evaluation of Pediatric Sleep Disorders

As is the case with other medical and psychiatric disorders, the key issue in evaluating pediatric sleep disorders is differential diagnosis. Because many sleep disorders present with similar symptomatology (e.g., excessive daytime sleepiness can have multiple causes), differential diagnosis is especially critical in the assessment of sleep complaints. Differentiation between a sleep disorder and other medical or psychological problems that may present with similar symptoms is also important. For example, a child with apparent night terrors may actually have a nocturnal seizure disorder. Similarly, what appears to be delayed sleep onset related to normal developmental nighttime fears may be a manifestation in some children of a more serious generalized anxiety disorder.

Furthermore, in many cases, two or more sleep disturbances may coexist, and medical and behavioral sleep disorders are frequently comorbid. For example, a child may have both obstructive sleep apnea and behavioral issues with bedtime refusal. Thus, treating the sleep apnea alone will alleviate nighttime arousals associated with sleep disordered breathing but will not eliminate bedtime resistance. In addition, the presence of one sleep problem may exacerbate another; for example, partial arousal parasomnias may be triggered by sleep deprivation in susceptible children. Finally, because sleep disorders can be secondary to physical illness or another psychological disorder, it is essential to evaluate for possible contributing factors to the sleep problem with a comprehensive and thorough history.

COMPONENTS OF THE PEDIATRIC SLEEP EVALUATION

An initial assessment of pediatric sleep disturbances typically includes (a) a sleep history, (b) a review of medical history, (c) a developmental screen/assessment of school functioning, (d) a family history, (e) a psychosocial history, (f) a behavioral assessment, and (g) a physical examina-

---

Dual Diagnoses in Sleep

There are a number of sleep disorders that are often related and frequently coexist:

- Obstructive sleep apnea–enuresis
- Obstructive sleep apnea–partial arousal parasomnias
- Chronic sleep deprivation–partial arousal parasomnias
- Insomnia–inadequate sleep hygiene
- Bedtime problems–nightwakings
- Restless legs syndrome–periodic limb movement disorder

---

tion. Further evaluation may include the completion of sleep diaries and/or an overnight polysomnogram or other diagnostic tests as appropriate. The sleep questionnaire presented below outlines a diagnostic approach that is generally appropriate across all age groups, from newborn through adolescence. (Focused questions pertaining to specific sleep disorders, such as obstructive sleep apnea and sleepwalking, are presented in the appropriate corresponding chapters.) Symptom-based algorithms also are provided in Chapter 5 to facilitate a basic approach to diagnosis and subsequent treatment. In addition, a sleep evaluation intake questionnaire is provided in Appendix A.

SLEEP HISTORY

Key Sleep Questions

1. Does your child have any problems going to bed?
2. Does your child have any problems falling asleep?
3. Does your child maintain a regular sleep schedule?
4. Does your child seem sleepy during the day and/or is it difficult to awaken your child in the morning?
5. Does your child wake up during the night?
6. Does your child have any unusual behaviors during the night?
7. Does your child snore or have any problems breathing during the night?

The first step in evaluating a child or adolescent for a sleep disorder is the completion of a thorough sleep history (including presenting complaint, sleep patterns and schedules, nocturnal behaviors, and symptoms of daytime sleepiness):

Presenting Complaint

All family members should describe the presenting complaint, especially the child/adolescent (if appropriate). Often differences in child/parent perception emerge, as well as differences in perception of the issues between parents. For example, parents may attribute sleep onset delay following lights out to non-compliance, whereas the child may state that he or she is "not sleepy" at the regular bedtime but can fall asleep easily an hour later. Included in the description of the presenting complaint should be a review of the onset, duration, and night-to-night consistency of the current sleep problem. A history of events that seem to have immediately preceded the onset of the sleep problem should also be elicited.

Sleep Patterns, Sleep Schedules, and Sleep Habits

No matter what the presenting sleep complaint, it is important to have a general sense of sleep patterns and behaviors. A review of sleep habits will often shed considerable light on the nature and cause of the presenting sleep complaint, and may also illuminate the presence of coexisting sleep problems and maladaptive sleep behaviors (inadequate sleep hygiene). General sleep behaviors over the previous several weeks (or over an average week, if the most recent weeks have been atypical) should be reviewed.

Bedtime

It is often easiest to have the family describe events from dinnertime until sleep onset in order to obtain a complete picture of bedtime behaviors. Specific information that may be helpful in elucidating the causes of and contributing factors to sleep problems include the following:

Bedtime schedule
- **Bedtime** (e.g., 8:00 PM)
- **Presence of a bedtime**, as some children are allowed to go to bed whenever they fall asleep rather than at a set time.
- **Time** of initiating the bedtime routine (time the child/adolescent begins to get ready for bed), time of lights out, and time of sleep onset (time the child actually falls asleep). Specifying these time periods may narrow the sleep problem down and help differentiate between bedtime resistance and difficulty falling asleep.

- **Consistency of bedtime** night-to-night, particularly weekday/weekend discrepancies.
- **Appropriateness of the bedtime** related to the child's natural or circadian fall-asleep time.
- **Supervision of bedtime** and whether the child or the parents typically decide when bedtime occurs.
- **The level of sleepiness** ("readiness" for bed) of the child at bedtime.

Bedtime routines
- **Evening activities,** particularly the child's involvement in stimulating evening activities, including television viewing, outside play, and videogames.
- **Presence of a bedtime routine,** that is, a series of consistent nighttime activities set up by parent and child leading to bedtime.
- **Duration of the bedtime routine,** as extended or elaborate routines lasting longer than 30 minutes may indicate a limit-setting problem.
- **Specific nature of the bedtime routine activities** and appropriateness for age. Also assess if these activities are likely to be stimulating for that child (e.g., baths are not relaxing for all children; in addition, the activity closest to bedtime should be the most soothing).
- **Location of the bedtime routine,** such as in the child's room versus the parents' room.
- **Television,** including the prominence of television viewing in the bedtime routine and presence of a television set in the child's bedroom.

Sleep associations. Sleep associations are behaviors that occur at the time of sleep initiation (e.g., nursing, rocking). Negative sleep associations can contribute to bedtime difficulties and nightwakings since behaviors that occur at bedtime (e.g., nursing, rocking) may be required to reinitiate sleep following normal nighttime arousals.

Bedtime stalling or refusal behaviors. A review of noncompliant behaviors should be conducted, including *types* of behaviors (e.g., crying, climbing out of crib, leaving room); *intensity* of the behaviors (e.g., calling out versus tantrums); *frequency* (how often they occur in a week period), and *duration* (how long they typically last), as well as the presence of bedtime fears. It is also important to assess any discrepancy between the child's behavior with one parent versus the other, and/or with other caretakers, as well as the parental reaction to the child's behavior at bedtime, including appropriateness of parents' response to bedtime behaviors (see also Chapter 6).

Falling asleep
- **Duration of time** between lights out and fall-asleep time.
- **Sleep onset location,** particularly where sleep onset typically occurs (e.g., living room) and the child's activity at the time (e.g., on the couch watching TV), and *variability* in location of sleep onset from night to night.
- **Transfers after sleep onset,** that is, whether the child falls asleep elsewhere and is subsequently transferred to his or her own bed.

Sleeping environment

- **Bedroom space and location,** including *bedroom sharing* with a parent, sibling, or other household member [some research indicates increased nightwakings in infants and toddlers who share a room with a parent(s)], and location of child's bedroom in relation to parents' room (e.g., child's anxiety may be increased if the bedroom is far away or on a different floor).
- **Light,** including use of nightlights and other lights in the room (child's need for bright lighting may be indicative of anxiety issues). Other sources of ambient light (e.g., streetlights; early morning eastern light) may interfere with normal circadian rhythm patterns.
- **Noise,** including amount and type of noise from other family members and outdoor noise, and sound levels at bedtime, during the night, and in the early morning.
- **Bed type,** as a crib provides natural limits to bedtime behaviors, a bed allows unlimited movement. Moving a child to a bed prematurely sometimes initiates or exacerbates sleep problems.

Co-sleeping, including assessment of intensity (all-night versus part-night co-sleeping), frequency (nightly versus intermittently), reasons for co-sleeping (lifestyle choice versus "reactive" co-sleeping in response to a sleep problem), and parents' reaction to co-sleeping (discrepancies in parent response).

Sleep Schedule

Naps, including timing and duration of naps, as well as ease or difficulty of falling asleep at naptime. It should be emphasized that unplanned naps at all ages and planned naps in a child older than 5 years is suggestive of inadequate sleep or an underlying sleep-disrupting factor.

Regularity of the sleep–wake schedule

- *Weekday schedule versus weekend schedule*, primarily the consistency of the sleep–wake schedule. In addition, it is particularly important in older children and adolescents to note the presence of *weekend oversleep*, as a total of 2 hours or more sleep on weekends compared to weeknights is indicative of inadequate sleep during the week.
- *Night-to-night* variability of the sleep schedule.
- *Daily schedule*, including timing of meals (e.g., too close to bedtime) and the regularity and structure of daytime activities (e.g., lack of exercise or timing of exercise periods near expected sleep onset).

Nocturnal Behaviors

Nighttime behaviors are important to review in order to obtain a complete picture of the sleep problem. These include *nightwakings* (including number and duration of nightwakings, behaviors that occur upon waking, parental response to nightwaking, and the manner in which the child returns to sleep, such as by nursing or with parental presence; see Chapter 7), the presence of *episodic* nocturnal events such as partial arousal parasomnias (see Chapter 10) and nightmares (see Chapter 9), as well as symptoms possibly suggestive of *sleep-disordered breathing* (see Chapter 13).

Daytime Behaviors

It is critical that daytime behaviors, particularly those that may be contributing to or indicative of significant daytime sleepiness (morning waking, daytime sleepiness and/or low functioning, and fatigue), be assessed in order to quantify the impact of the sleep disturbance on the child and family.

Morning awakening
- **Time of awakening,** including weekday to weekend discrepancy and time child spontaneously awakens, or would spontaneously awaken if allowed.
- **Mood** upon awakening, such as irritable and groggy versus alert and "ready to start the day."
- **Difficulty waking** in the morning, including need for multiple attempts at waking by parents, siblings, or others. Difficulty waking in the morning in conjunction with an adequate sleep schedule is indicative of an underlying sleep-disrupting factor (e.g., sleep disordered breathing, periodic limb movement disorder).
- **Consequences of difficulty waking,** including habitual tardiness or school absences.

You Snooze, You Lose

In general, the habitual need for an alarm clock in order to awaken in the morning, especially multiple "snooze alarm" hits, strongly suggests insufficient sleep. This is particularly true in school-aged children, who should awaken spontaneously in the morning if adequately rested.

Daytime sleepiness. Falling asleep in school, while riding in a car, or during other activities is indicative of inadequate sleep or an underlying sleep disruption. In younger children, daytime sleepiness may be manifested as "overtiredness," with the child overactive and engaging in problem behaviors.

Daytime functioning. Inadequate or poor sleep may have negative consequences on a host of functional domains, including mood, behavior, attention, learning, school performance, social relationships, and health.

Fatigue/tiredness. Sleepiness is the tendency to doze off or fall asleep, often in inappropriate settings, and generally implies insufficient and/or disrupted sleep. Complaints of fatigue or being tired, on the other hand, are often indicative of subjective feelings of low energy and low motivation, which may or may not be primarily a result of poor sleep. Fatigue is defined as lethargy without sleep initiation, and tends to be associated with medical (e.g., thyroid function) or psychiatric (e.g., depression) disorders. However, a distinction between sleepiness and fatigue is not always possible, as there may be considerable overlap in descriptions of these two states by parents and/or older children and adolescents.

MEDICAL HISTORY

A standard pediatric medical history and review of systems should be elicited, with particular emphasis on past and current medical conditions, prior hospitalizations and surgeries (especially prior history of adenotonsillectomy for symptoms of sleep disordered breathing), and medications (see Chapter 19 for a complete review of the effects of specific medications on sleep).

DEVELOPMENTAL/SCHOOL HISTORY

A developmental history is important, including a history of developmental disabilities, prematurity, and impaired neurologic functioning, as there is often an increased prevalence of sleep problems in children with developmental delays (see Chapter 20). Academic problems are one of the most important sequelae of insufficient and/or disrupted sleep. Furthermore, a developmental history and assessment of academic functioning in school-aged children will help provide a context for the current sleep difficulties.

FAMILY HISTORY

A family history of sleep problems can be helpful in confirming the diagnosis of certain sleep disorders, especially for those disorders that may have a genetic component. Such diagnoses include partial arousal parasomnias (sleep terrors and sleepwalking), restless legs syndrome, obstructive sleep apnea, and narcolepsy. In many cases, these disorders have not been formally diagnosed in family members, but symptoms are clearly present if directly questioned ("His father snores so loudly, he has to sleep in another room!"). In addition, parental experience with sleep problems, such as chronic insomnia, may impact on parental attitudes toward and management of similar sleep problems in the child.

Like Father, Like Son

One of the most rewarding aspects of diagnosing and treating pediatric sleep disorders is the potential to impact the whole family. Not only does successful treatment of a child's sleep problem result in everyone getting a better night's sleep, but it may encourage adult family members to obtain needed help for their own sleep problems. Parents may be much more willing to seek medical attention for loud snoring, daytime sleepiness, or symptoms of restless legs when their child is also being evaluated and treated for a similar symptom.

PSYCHOSOCIAL HISTORY

A complete psychosocial history is appropriate, including the following:

- **Family functioning,** including overall family functioning; effectiveness of parenting skills (including limit setting); family structure (e.g., siblings, extended family members in household, one-parent versus two-parent household); parental psychological functioning (e.g., parental depression); and family discord.
- **Parental separation or divorce,** including time elapsed since the separation or divorce, visitation schedules and level of involvement of noncustodial parent, consistency of sleep patterns and habits across households, discrepancies in parenting styles, and stress on the child.
- **Significant life events,** such as death of a family member, change in school, or a recent move, that may result in adjustment sleep problems.
- **Family and cultural context,** including ethnic influences on sleep behaviors, family values regarding health priorities, and family beliefs about sleep and importance of sleep.
- **Impact on family** of the sleep problem, including the effect of the child's sleep on the parents' sleep, impact on parents' daytime functioning, and impact on marital satisfaction.

BEHAVIORAL ASSESSMENT

A behavioral/psychological assessment is important because sleep disturbances can result in psychiatric symptoms, such as mood changes and oppositional behavior; conversely, psychiatric disorders can result in sleep disturbances. Thus, particularly in older children and adolescents, it is important to elicit possible symptoms of depression, anxiety, and other psychiatric disorders.

PHYSICAL EXAMINATION

A physical exam should be conducted on all children and adolescents being evaluated for sleep complaints. Although the physical examination is noncontributory for many sleep disorders in children, careful attention should be paid to the following specific points:

- **Growth parameters,** including height, weight, and age-adjusted body mass index. For example, growth failure and obesity/overweight are both associated both sleep disordered breathing.
- **General appearance,** including activity level and evidence of fatigue and/or sleepiness. Children with severe obstructive sleep apnea or significant sleep deprivation may actually doze off in the office setting.
- **Otolaryngologic exam,** including examination of the nose, mouth, and throat for possible risk factors (e.g., adenotonsillar hypertrophy) for suspected obstructive sleep apnea (see Chapter 13). The HEENT (head, eyes, ears, nose, throat) exam may also suggest evidence of atopic disease contributing to sleep disordered breathing.
- **Neurologic assessment.** Particular attention should be paid to the neurologic examination in cases where the concern is excessive sleepiness or where there is a possibility of nocturnal seizures.

SLEEP DIARIES

An important step in the evaluation of sleep problems is the collection of sleep diaries. A typical sleep diary includes information on time to bed, latency to sleep onset, number and duration of nighttime awakenings, time of waking, total sleep time, and duration and time of naps. Two weeks of baseline sleep diaries is usually adequate to delineate sleep patterns (samples of different styles of sleep diaries are provided in Appendix B). In older school-aged children and adolescents, the patient can usually complete the sleep diaries, which can foster independence and ownership of sleep behaviors.

OVERNIGHT POLYSOMNOGRAPHY

Once basic information regarding the sleep history as well as a review of medical, developmental, and behavioral issues have been obtained, it is important to determine whether an overnight sleep study ("polysomnography") is needed. A polysomnogram (PSG) is a diagnostic tool that outlines sleep architecture and shows details about breathing, body movements, and arousals during sleep. Many sleep disorders centers require an initial evaluation in a sleep clinic before a sleep study can be scheduled, whereas other sleep laboratories will take direct referrals from primary care physicians if adequate documentation of the problem and the need for a sleep study is made available.

When Is a PSG Warranted?

A PSG is warranted principally to diagnose sleep disordered breathing, especially obstructive sleep apnea; to investigate sleep-related causes of excessive daytime sleepiness, such as narcolepsy or sleep fragmentation due to frequent nocturnal arousals (including periodic limb movement disorder); and occasionally to delineate the etiology of episodic nocturnal phenomena (e.g., parasomnias versus nocturnal seizures).

Indications for ordering an overnight PSG include the following:

- **Sleep disordered breathing.** To document the presence and severity of sleep disordered breathing (obstructive sleep apnea). In addition, follow-up testing after an adenotonsillectomy may be necessary (see Chapter 13).
- **Continuous positive airway pressure (CPAP) or bilevel positive airway pressure (BiPAP).** To titrate for CPAP or BiPAP pressure in the treatment of sleep disordered breathing (see Chapter 13).
- **Limb movements.** To assess for abnormal limb movements (periodic limb movement disorder; see Chapter 14) and any associated sleep fragmentation.
- **Episodic nocturnal phenomena.** To evaluate episodic nocturnal phenomena, such as parasomnias, that are frequent, violent, atypical, prolonged, or resistant to treatment. However, it should be kept in mind that a single overnight sleep study may fail to capture an event, given the sporadic nature of many parasomnias. In this situation, asking the parent to videotape an event in the home setting may yield more information and be more cost effective.
- **Unexplained daytime sleepiness.** Disruptions in sleep architecture may reflect primary abnormalities that are part of a sleep disorder (narcolepsy). These disruptions may also be secondary to sleep fragmentation or deprivation.

The standard overnight PSG involves recording a number of different parameters during sleep with close monitoring by a qualified technician. The following parameters are usually recorded: *respiratory effort* (chest wall and abdominal motion using piezo crystal belts), *ventilation* (end-tidal PCO_2 sampled at the nose and/or mouth or transcutaneous CO_2), *airflow* (oral and nasal thermisters or capnography), *heart rate* (ECG, typically modified lead II), *respiratory rate*, hemoglobin *oxygen saturation* (pulse oximeter), *sleep staging* [electroencephalogram (EEG), electromyogram of chin (EMG), and electro-oculogram (EOG)], *arousals* (EEG), *leg movements* (anterior tibialis EMG), *snoring* (microphone), and *body movements* (video recording). A sample polysomnography montage and 30-second epoch is presented in Fig. 4.1,

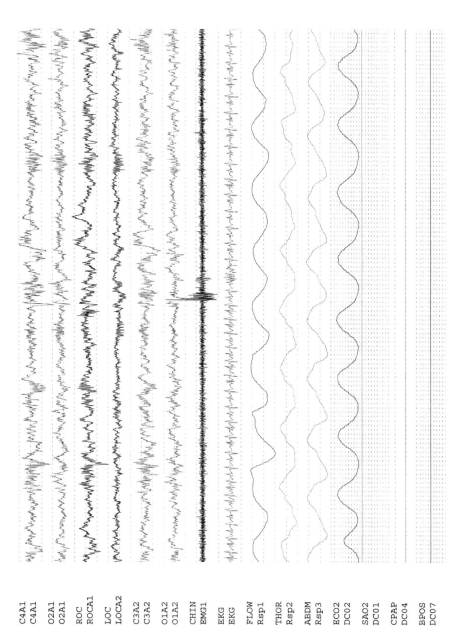

C4A1
C4A1

O2A1
O2A1

ROC
ROCA1

LOC
LOCA2

C3A2
C3A2

O1A2
O1A2

CHIN
EMG1

EKG
EKG

FLOW
Rsp1

THOR
Rsp2

ABDM
Rsp3

ECO2
DC02

SAO2
DC01

CPAP
DC04

BPOS
DC07

FIG. 4.1. Pediatric polysomnography montage. C4A1, O2A1, C3A2, O1A2: EEG leads; ROC: right eye; LOC: left eye; FLOW: nasal airflow; THOR: thoracic movement; ABDM: abdominal movement; ECO2: end-tidal CO_2; SAO2: oxygen saturation; BPOS: body position.

which is representative of a standard pediatric recording montage used by most sleep laboratories. Some pediatric studies may include additional EEG leads.

Some laboratories measure esophageal pressures with transesophageal balloon manometry for evaluation of upper airway resistance syndrome (see Chapter 13), but this is not done routinely. It should be noted that some sleep labs use only two central and two occipital electroencephalographic channels and, thus, do not provide a full EEG montage; therefore, if seizures are a diagnostic consideration, a separate evaluation may be necessary.

Most overnight studies are done in the lab, although home studies are sometimes used. Lab studies have the benefit of increased validity and inclusion of behavioral observation. In addition, both home and nap studies have a high false-negative rate for sleep disordered breathing.

An overnight PSG can be performed in a child of any age or in a child with an underlying chronic illness if adequately trained staff and appropriate equipment are used. A child-friendly environment is ideal in order to facilitate a good night's sleep and to minimize the anxiety associated with an unfamiliar environment. Sedation is not recommended for a sleep study, as most sedating agents are also respiratory depressants. Young children are accompanied by one parent throughout the night but sleep in a separate bed. In preparation for the study, it is preferable to provide a tour of the sleep lab. It is important also to notify the sleep laboratory of any special considerations involved with the children being evaluated, such as anxiety, fears, and medications.

Pediatric sleep studies should be scored and interpreted by technicians and physicians who have specific training in pediatric sleep medicine, using age-appropriate criteria defined by the American Thoracic Society consensus statement. The limitations inherent in using polysomnography are the shortage of facilities that perform pediatric studies and interpretation using age-appropriate criteria. The interpretation of PSGs in beyond the scope of this discussion, as it requires considerable experience and detailed evaluation of the data.

Additional studies. As an adjunct to a nocturnal PSG, a *multiple sleep latency test* (MSLT) may be conducted to objectively evaluate an individual's level of daytime sleepiness and sleep onset structure (see Chapter 15). Adult norms for "pathologic" levels of sleepiness are generally applied to adolescents, but no widely accepted norms for children currently exist. The MSLT consists of four or five 20-minute nap opportunities given at 2-hour intervals on the morning following an overnight sleep study. The basic parameters measured are *latency to sleep onset* (if sleep does occurs within each of the 20-minute nap opportunities, which are then averaged over the four or five naps to yield a *mean sleep onset latency)* and *latency to REM sleep.* Mean sleep onset latency on MSLT in adults is considered to be pathologic if less than 5 minutes, possibly abnormal if between 5 and 10 minutes, and normal if greater than 10 minutes. In school-aged children, a normal mean sleep onset latency is considered to be about 16 to 18 minutes; children in this age range with a mean sleep onset latency of less than 16 minutes are considered at risk for having significant daytime sleepiness. Sleep onset in three or more naps and/or the presence of frequent "microsleeps" (<30-second epochs of sleep) on the MSLT are also highly suggestive of abnormal levels of sleepiness. Pathologic levels of sleepiness are generally associated with narcolepsy but may also occur as a reflection of significant chronic sleep deprivation. A very short REM sleep onset latency (also known as sleep onset REM periods or SOREMPs) may occur with profound sleep loss however it can be indicative of narcolepsy. Consultation with a sleep specialist is recommended for interpretation of the MSLT.

5

Symptom-Based Algorithms

The following algorithms present a clinical framework for evaluating three of the most common presenting sleep complaints in pediatrics (bedtime resistance/prolonged sleep onset, night wakings, and daytime sleepiness in adolescents). The major diagnostic categories to consider for each presenting complaint are printed in bold; important differentiating features are outlined in italics; and suggested diagnostic tests are underlined. It is important to keep in mind that there may be more than one etiology for a sleep complaint in any given child or adolescent; thus, several diagnostic categories may need to be considered. In addition, children may present with more than one sleep complaint (e.g., delayed sleep onset and night wakings). Finally, these algorithms represent only a *guideline* for clinical evaluation. Specific assessment, diagnostic, and treatment recommendations for each disorder are found within the individual chapters.

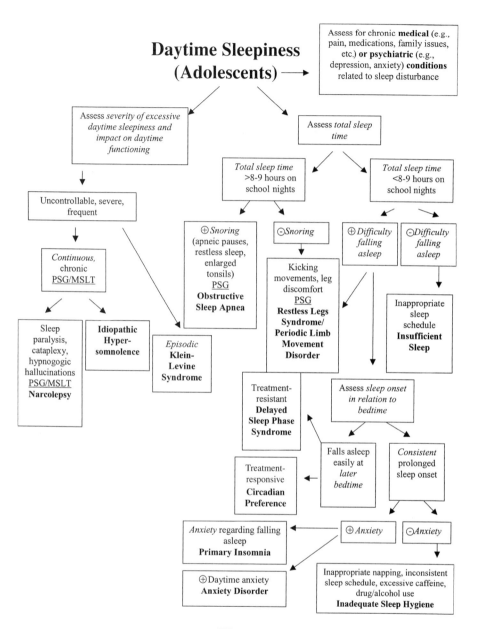

FIG. 5.1

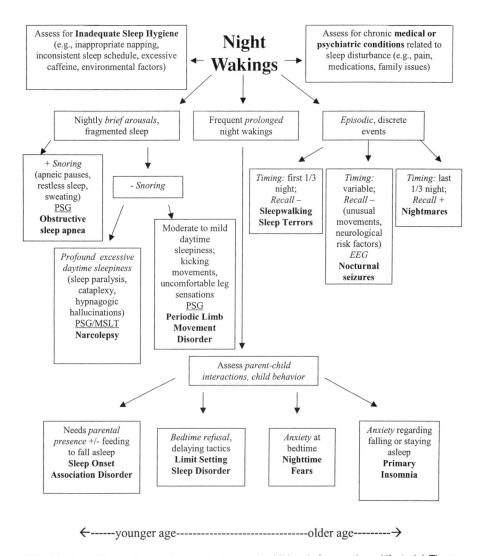

FIG. 5.2. Note: The etiology of sleep disturbances in children is frequently multifactorial. Therefore, any evaluation of nightwakings should take into consideration all of the factors listed above.

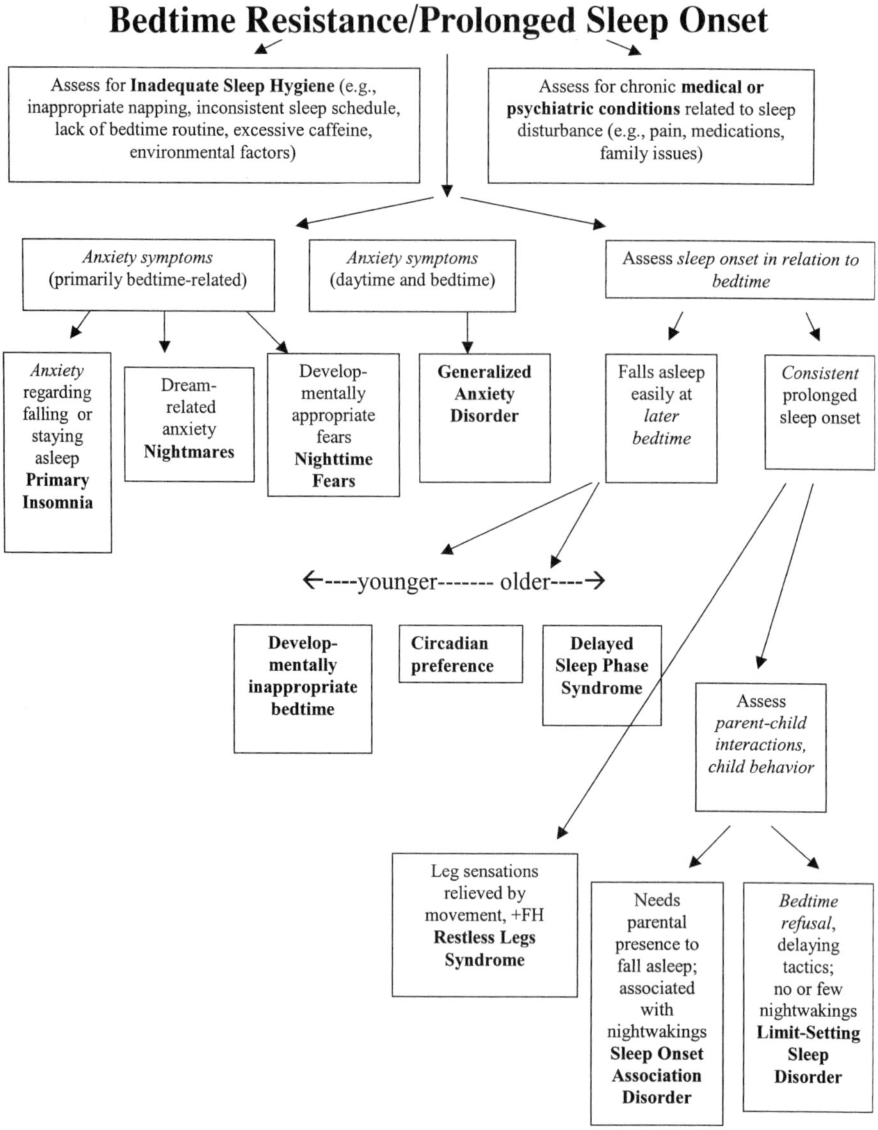

Bedtime Resistance/Prolonged Sleep Onset

Assess for **Inadequate Sleep Hygiene** (e.g., inappropriate napping, inconsistent sleep schedule, lack of bedtime routine, excessive caffeine, environmental factors)

Assess for chronic **medical or psychiatric conditions** related to sleep disturbance (e.g., pain, medications, family issues)

Anxiety symptoms (primarily bedtime-related)

Anxiety symptoms (daytime and bedtime)

Assess *sleep onset in relation to bedtime*

Anxiety regarding falling or staying asleep **Primary Insomnia**

Dream-related anxiety **Nightmares**

Developmentally appropriate fears **Nighttime Fears**

Generalized Anxiety Disorder

Falls asleep easily at *later bedtime*

Consistent prolonged sleep onset

←----younger------- older----→

Developmentally inappropriate bedtime

Circadian preference

Delayed Sleep Phase Syndrome

Assess *parent-child interactions, child behavior*

Leg sensations relieved by movement, +FH **Restless Legs Syndrome**

Needs parental presence to fall asleep; associated with nightwakings **Sleep Onset Association Disorder**

Bedtime refusal, delaying tactics; no or few nightwakings **Limit-Setting Sleep Disorder**

FIG. 5.3

6

Bedtime Problems

Bedtime problems, including stalling and refusing to go to bed, are often the result of parental difficulties in setting limits and managing behavior. Sleep disturbances of this type generally fall within the diagnostic category known as *limit-setting sleep disorder*. These sleep problems typically begin after the age of 2 years, when children are either able to climb out of the crib or have been moved to a bed. *Bedtime stalling* behaviors include attempts to delay bedtime (e.g., by watching additional television) or the bedtime routine (e.g., by reading another story), or occur following lights out ("curtain calls," such as requests for a drink of water or an additional hug). Typically, the requests are based on what the child has learned will elicit a parental response, whether that is a trip to the bathroom or being "afraid" of monsters under the bed. *Bedtime refusal* includes behaviors such as the child refusing to get ready for bed or refusing to remain in the bed or the bedroom, often following the parent(s) back to the living room or other room of the house.

Limit-Setting Sleep Disorder

Limit-setting sleep disorder is characterized by the inadequate enforcement of bedtime limits by a caretaker, with resultant stalling or refusal to go to bed at an appropriate time. When limits (bedtimes) are not set and enforced or are enforced only sporadically, sleep will be delayed, and total sleep may not be enough to meet the child's sleep needs.

Another type of limit-setting problem occurs when there are few or no limits instituted at all by parents around sleep behaviors; examples include allowing the child to fall asleep while watching television in the living room or allowing an older child to play computer games in his or her bedroom. Parents may also institute limits in an unpredictable or inconsistent way (e.g., intermittently allowing the child to fall asleep in the parents' bed). This type of inconsistent parental response provides intermittent reinforcement and maintains the behavior. Limit-setting sleep problems may also affect parental response to nightwakings, as in the case of the child who is allowed to join the parents in their bed during the night. Parental limit-setting is also likely to be the problem if the child goes to bed and falls asleep quickly for others (e.g., babysitter, other parent) or has no difficulty falling asleep at the desired bedtime in other situations (e.g., allowed to stay in living room and falls asleep on couch watching television).

The environment may also contribute to limit-setting problems. For example, limits may be difficult to set in homes in which the child shares a bedroom with his or her parents or siblings. Parents of children with a current or past history of medical problems may also have difficulty setting limits, because of guilt, a sense that the child is "vulnerable," or concerns about doing psychological harm (see Chapter 21 for more information on children with medical problems).

EPIDEMIOLOGY

Bedtime resistance, found in 10% to 30% of toddlers and preschoolers, is one of the most common concerns of parents and may coexist with nightwakings. Not only are bedtime problems common, but this behaviorally based sleep problem often becomes chronic; in one study, 84% of children aged 15 to 48 months with bedtime struggles and/or nightwaking continued to have significant sleep disturbance at 3-year follow-up. School-aged children may also have significant limit-setting sleep issues; in one study, 15% of children aged 4 to 10 years had problematic bedtime resistance reported by parents.

ETIOLOGY/RISK FACTORS

- **Permissive parenting style** in which there is minimal limit-setting regarding most discipline issues.
- **Conflicting parental discipline styles,** especially when parents frequently disagree about how to handle behavioral issues. In this situation, one parent is often the authoritarian, whereas the other is more lenient ("good cop/bad cop"). Children often sense (and sometimes exploit) this ambivalence, leading to increased noncompliant behavior.
- **Age,** as toddlers and preschool-aged children are more likely to assert their independence and refuse to comply with parental requests. As children get older, they typically require less parental interaction at bedtime.
- **Temperament,** especially difficult and unpredictable temperament styles.
- **Oppositional behavior** during the day, which makes noncompliance at bedtime more likely.
- **Environmental settings** that inhibit limit-setting, such as parents and child sharing a bedroom or living with grandparents.

It should be noted that circadian timing may also play a role in some cases of bedtime struggles. When a relatively early bedtime coincides with the normal late-day circadian-mediated surge in alertness (otherwise known as a "second wind"), a child may have significantly more difficulty settling and this can result in bedtime resistance. Children with an "owl" circadian preference for later sleep onset and wake times also tend to have a later circadian nadir and are, thus, particularly likely to have a settling problem if bedtime is set too early. These children may also resist going to bed because they are not ready to fall asleep at the parent-determined bedtime. These situations are not primarily caused by parental failure to set limits, but the resulting sleep onset problems may be compounded by parental management.

PRESENTATION/SYMPTOMS

- **Noncompliant behavior** in response to parental requests to get ready for bed (e.g., change into pajamas, brush teeth).
- **Bedtime resistance,** including refusal to go to bed or requiring a parent to be present at bedtime.
- **"Curtain calls,"** characterized by frequent requests for parental attention (e.g., drinks, kisses) after lights out
- **Delayed sleep onset** of 30 minutes or more following lights out.

Diagnostic Criteria

See Table 6.1.

Associated Features

- **Nightwakings.** Many children with bedtime struggles also present with frequent nightwakings, resulting from similar limit-setting issues or as a result of negative sleep associations (e.g., parental presence required to fall asleep) that have developed at bedtime (see Chapter 7).

TABLE 6.1. *Diagnostic criteria: limit-setting sleep disorder (307.42)*

A. The patient has difficulty initiating sleep.
B. The patient stalls or refuses to go to bed at an appropriate time.
C. Once the sleep period is initiated, sleep is of normal quality and duration.
D. Polysomnographic monitoring demonstrates normal timing, quality, and duration of the sleep period.
E. No significant underlying mental or medical disorder accounts for the complaint.
F. The symptoms do not meet criteria for any other sleep disorder causing difficulty in initiating sleep (e.g., sleep-onset association disorder).

Minimal criteria: B plus C.
Used with permission from American Academy of Sleep Medicine. *The international classification of sleep disorders, revised: diagnostic and coding manual.* Westchester, IL: AASM, 1997: 93–94.

- **"Fearful behaviors."** Some children present with nighttime fears characterized by fearful behaviors (e.g., crying, clinging, leaving bedroom to seek parental reassurance) that are a manifestation of bedtime stalling rather than anxiety based.
- **Daytime behavior problems.** Daytime behavior problems appear to be more common in "poor sleepers." This relationship may reflect an increase in behavior problems because of inadequate sleep or may be related to the fact that children with daytime behavior problems are more likely to have similar problems at night, or a combination of both.
- **Family tension.** Bedtime resistance often results in significant family tension, including arguments between the child and the parents, and marital discord. This tension may contribute to heightened arousal in the child, making sleep onset even more difficult. Parents also may focus more attention on the child's behavior at bedtime to avoid dealing with underlying marital conflicts.

EVALUATION

- **Medical history:** Generally benign. Children with medical conditions may be more likely to have bedtime struggles, related to a number of physical (pain, medication) and behavioral issues (see Chapter 21).
- **Developmental history:** Developmentally delayed children and children with sensory integration issues may have more difficulty with self-soothing at bedtime.
- **Family history:** Should include an evaluation of parenting skills and limit-setting abilities.
- **Behavioral assessment:** A history of more global behavior problems, especially noncompliance and oppositional defiant disorder (ODD), may be present. Children with attention deficit-hyperactivity disorder (ADHD) often have more difficulty settling at bedtime (see Chapter 22).
- **Physical examination:** Usually noncontributory.
- **Diagnostic tests:** Not indicated.

DIFFERENTIAL DIAGNOSIS

Bedtime struggles may be the result of a more global problem with noncompliance, including ODD. In addition, alternative reasons for delayed sleep onset should be considered:

- **Inappropriate sleep schedules** may contribute to delayed sleep onset. Naps, including napping past 4:00 PM or continued napping in an older preschooler, may result in a later sleep onset. In addition, an irregular sleep schedule (inconsistent bedtime and waketime) may conflict with the circadian sleep–wake rhythm and contribute to difficulties in falling asleep. Similarly, significant discrepancies between weekday and weekend sleep schedules can result in problems falling asleep on Sunday evenings, especially if the child or adolescent is sleeping in late on weekend mornings. Finally, parents may not be attentive to the child's natural sleep onset time, which may be later than the desired bedtime.

Nap Problems

Parents of young children often struggle with naptime issues. Similar to bedtime problems and nightwakings (see Chapter 7), nap problems are often related to scheduling problems and/or poor sleep associations. To deal with naptime problems, the following strategies can be beneficial:

- **Set naptimes** that are either based on the same time each day (e.g., 9:00 AM and 1:00 PM) or occur within 2 to 3 hours after the last awakening. Up to the age of 6 to 9 months, most babies are ready to take a nap exactly 2 hours after awakening.
- **Set a consistent naptime routine** that is similar to, but shorter than, the bedtime routine. For children who are taking only one nap per day, have the nap occur immediately following lunch so that there is a clear routine to the day.
- **Develop positive sleep habits,** including self-soothing skills. Similar to nightwakings, an infant or toddler who develops negative sleep associations (e.g., being rocked to sleep) will require this to occur at the onset of the nap and will be unable to return to sleep following a brief arousal. Negative sleep associations often account for babies who only nap for a short period, e.g., 20 to 45 minutes.
- **Establish clear naptime rules,** especially with toddlers.

- **Delayed sleep phase,** related to an "owl" tendency or, in some cases, delayed sleep phase syndrome (see Chapter 16). In both situations, sleep onset occurs at a consistent time each night, and no problems are noted if bedtime is set closer to the usual fall-asleep time.
- **Nighttime fears,** in which anxiety is a significant component of the child's bedtime behavior. Typically, if the parents remain with an anxious child at bedtime, resistance disappears and sleep onset is not delayed.
- **Transient insomnia,** which is likely to present in children with previously normal sleep. Transient insomnia can be the result of sleeping in an unfamiliar or nonconducive (e.g., too noisy, too hot) sleep environment; stressful life event; disruption of sleep schedule (e.g., trip, jet lag); or illness.
- **Restless legs syndrome** often presents with difficulty falling asleep at bedtime. Restless legs syndrome is characterized by uncomfortable sensations and increased movements in the legs that interfere with sleep onset (see Chapter 14).

- **Medication effects,** including stimulant medications for ADHD, may result in delayed sleep onset (see Chapter 19 for more information on medication effects).

MANAGEMENT

When to Refer

Children or adolescents with persistent or severe bedtime issues that are not responsive to simple behavioral measures or which are extremely disruptive should be referred to a mental health professional for evaluation and treatment. Collaboration with a behavioral therapist in designing and implementing treatment plans may be prudent if there are complex, chronic, or multiple sleep problems, or if initial behavioral strategies have failed.

Impact on the Family

Successful behavioral intervention for bedtime resistance will not only result in improvement in the child's sleep problems, but is also likely to alleviate parental stress and improve parental sleep. Implementation of behavioral management strategies for sleep may also generalize to improvements in parenting skills and management of daytime behaviors.

Treatment

Treatment for limit-setting sleep problems should include the institution of appropriate sleep habits, development of an appropriate sleep schedule that coincides with the child's natural circadian rhythm, and appropriate and consistent parental limit-setting.

Sleep habits
- **Establish a set bedtime** that coincides with the child's natural sleep onset time. A consistent nightly bedtime will help to set the circadian clock and enable the child to fall asleep more easily. If, however, the attempted bedtime coincides with the late-day circadian peak in alertness, the likely result is bedtime resistance. In this case, delaying the bedtime, or moving the bedtime earlier, when the child is more physiologically ready for sleep, may be warranted. With children who have an evening circadian preference, temporarily delaying the bedtime to coincide with the natural sleep onset time and then gradually advancing the bedtime over a period of several weeks may be a reasonable approach (see discussion of bedtime fading, below).
- **Institute bedtime fading,** which involves temporarily setting the bedtime at the current sleep onset time and then gradually advancing it to the desired

bedtime. This has the advantage of temporarily eliminating the struggles that occur between bedtime and sleep onset, thus reducing tension in the household. In addition, children usually view this procedure positively (being "allowed" to stay up later), which increases the likelihood of compliance with the rest of the behavioral program.

- **Evaluate daytime sleep habits,** particularly in older children, that may be interfering with sleep onset, such as napping. Preschoolers often continue to require a daytime nap, but daytime sleep past 3:00 or 4:00 in the afternoon interferes with an early bedtime. In these cases, bedtimes need to be moved later and parental expectations need to be adjusted.
- **Establish a consistent bedtime routine** that is approximately 20 to 45 minutes and includes three or four soothing activities (e.g., bath, pajamas, stories) rather than high-energy or stimulating activities (e.g., playing outside, watching television). The final activity (e.g., stories) should be a preferred one to motivate compliance with prior activities (e.g., brushing teeth). A chart of the bedtime routine can be highly beneficial.
- **Provide a transitional object,** such as a blanket, doll, or stuffed animal.
- **Maintain good sleep hygiene practices,** such as avoiding caffeine and getting regular exercise.

Behavior Management Strategies

Bedtime problems are similar to any other behavioral issue and, thus, respond to general behavior management strategies. Suggestions for parents include the following:

- **Use positive reinforcement** to increase appropriate behaviors.
- **Avoid punishment** to decrease inappropriate behaviors, as punishment is not an effective way to change a child's behavior.
- **Focus on increasing positive behaviors** rather than decreasing negative behaviors.
- **Be consistent in responding,** as this is the key to behavior change.
- **Do not ask questions** (e.g., "Ready for bed?") when the intention is to provide a command (e.g., " Time for bed.").
- **Set clear limits and follow through.**
- **Provide acceptable choices** (e.g., " Do you want to now or in 5 minutes?") to give a child some control but within reasonable limits.

Limit-setting: guidelines for parents
- **Establish clear bedtime rules,** including activities involved in getting ready for bed (e.g., change into pajamas, brush teeth). Parents should also identify specific appropriate and inappropriate bedtime behaviors for the child (e.g., staying in bed, not calling for parents).

- **Ignore any complaints or protests** about bedtime (e.g., "I'm not tired," "I don't want to go to bed"). Parents should also avoid discussing or arguing about bedtime as this will lead to a struggle, often reinforcing bedtime problems with increased attention. Parents should firmly and calmly let their child know it is time for bed and continue with the established routine.
- **Put child to bed drowsy but awake,** as it is beneficial for children to learn to fall asleep independently.
- **Check on the child** if he or she is upset or crying. The visits should be brief (1 minute) and boring, and occur at a frequency that is comfortable for both parents and child. These "check-ins" provide reassurance, but at the same time should be structured to reinforce limits.
- **Return child to bed or room** firmly and calmly if he or she comes out of the bedroom. For some children, simply returning them to bed multiple times works. For others, establishing a system in which the bedroom door is closed for a brief period (1 minute) if the child gets out of bed can be helpful. The time can be increased by 1 minute for each successive time out of bed. In addition, parents should praise their child for positive behaviors (e.g., staying in bed, not calling).
- **Use positive reinforcement,** including sticker charts and reward systems. Small rewards should be given contingent on positive behaviors and, especially in younger children, rewards should be presented immediately (first thing in the morning). Larger rewards can be offered for continued positive behaviors, such as three nights of going to bed without protest. The specific behaviors and number of days/nights required to earn a reward should be based on the child's developmental level (younger children need more frequent rewards) and should be based on the number of successes rather than on number of consecutive nights of success (e.g., three stickers obtain a trip to the playground, *not* three consecutive stickers). The reward schedule should also be set up initially to ensure a reasonable expectation of immediate success, which is likely to increase the child's investment in the process.
- **Stick to firm bedtime limits** once clear rules have been established. Parents must follow through on their expectations and not inadvertently reinforce inappropriate behaviors.
- **Be persistent and consistent** in responding to the child. Consistency is the key to any behavior change. It is very important to explain to parents that *intermittent* reinforcement of an undesired behavior (occasionally allowing the child to fall asleep in the parent's bed) actually makes it *more difficult* to extinguish or eliminate the behavior. The analogy of "playing slot machines" may help parents understand this important behavioral concept; that is, the more unpredictable the reward is ("winning the jackpot" or "getting to stay in Mom's bed"), the more likely the individual is to persist in the behavior ("pulling the slot machine lever" or "coming into the bedroom").
- **Expect an "extinction burst"** after initiation of a behavioral program. It is very important to warn parents that the behavior will often become worse

(intensify in severity and frequency) for several days before significant improvement occurs. Anticipating this often prevents parents from immediately abandoning the behavioral program.

PROGNOSIS

Bedtime struggles can usually be well-controlled with behavioral interventions.

Tips for Talking to Parents

- **Explain the role of limit-setting** in bedtime stalling and bedtime refusal.
- **Discuss developmentally appropriate parental responses** to and strategies for handling noncompliant bedtime behaviors.
- **Develop an appropriate sleep schedule** that ensures adequate sleep and avoids sleep deprivation. Be sure the set bedtime is appropriate given the child's circadian rhythm and preference.
- **Develop a behavior management plan** that incorporates all potential pitfalls.
- **Refer for behavioral management** if the bedtime problems are indicative of more global parenting limitations or the bedtime problems are unresponsive to simple behavioral interventions.

See Appendix F1 for parent handout on bedtime problems.

7

Nightwakings

Nightwakings are one of the most common sleep problems experienced by infants and toddlers. By 6 months of age, most babies are physiologically capable of sleeping throughout the night and no longer require nighttime feedings. However, 25% to 50% continue to awaken during the night. Studies also indicate that nightwakings are likely to persist, as young children often do not "outgrow" the problem.

Nightwakings occur for many different reasons, but persistent and problematic nightwakings are commonly related to inappropriate sleep onset associations. Sleep onset associations are conditions that the child *learns to need* in order to fall asleep at bedtime. These same sleep onset associations are also often needed in order to fall *back to sleep* after arousals or awakenings during the night. Thus, when a child develops bedtime sleep onset associations that are not readily available during the night (being rocked or held, having parental presence), prolonged nightwakings may occur. As infants and children typically arouse briefly on average four to six times throughout the night as a result of the normal ultradian rhythm of sleep cycles, these nightwakings (or, more accurately, these failures to fall back to sleep) may occur as often as every 90–120 minutes.

Children who are able to soothe themselves back to sleep without parental intervention ("self-soothers") generally experience brief arousals rather than prolonged nightwakings. This capacity to self-soothe is clearly associated with the practice of being put to bed while drowsy but still awake (avoiding associating sleep onset with being held or rocked) and, thus, without sleep onset associations that will be unavailable during the night. Parents are generally unaware of these brief arousals. In contrast, "signalers" are those children who alert their parents by crying or going into the parents' bedroom upon awakening. Many of these signaler children have developed inappropriate sleep onset associations and, thus, have difficulty self-soothing. Parents, especially with infants and toddlers, then choose whether or not to respond to the signaled arousal/waking with such behaviors as verbal soothing, rocking, or feeding. The practice of parents immediately responding to signaled nightwakings, particularly if the interaction is reinforcing for the infant, may result in a "trained night crier."

Finally, it should be noted that there is often considerable night-to-night and week-to-week variability in all of these behaviors, and neither infants nor parents are always consistent in the way they behave and interact. However, it is clear that a pattern of persistent difficulty in self-soothing is associated with frequent and problematic nightwakings in infants.

Sleep Associations

Sleep associations are those conditions that are present at the time of sleep onset. These conditions are usually required again following normal nighttime arousals. They can be positive sleep associations (e.g., thumbsucking) or negative sleep associations (e.g., rocking, nursing, swinging). Negative sleep associations require parental intervention and cannot be reestablished by the child upon awakening during the night. Negative sleep associations are the primary cause of frequent wakings during the night.

EPIDEMIOLOGY

Studies indicate that 25%–50% of 6- to 12-month-olds and 30% of 1-year-olds have problematic nightwakings. In toddlers (aged 1–3 years), 15%–20% continue to have nightwakings.

ETIOLOGY/RISK FACTORS

As discussed above, the primary cause of frequent nightwakings is negative sleep associations. Children who experience more frequent arousals also have more opportunities to have nightwakings. Conditions that may increase the likelihood of arousal include:

- **Co-sleeping,** as studies have found that babies who either share a room or share a bed with their parent(s) are highly likely to awaken during the night and seek interaction with a parent.
- **Breast-feeding,** given that breast milk is more easily digested and breast-fed babies need to be fed more frequently. Breast-fed babies are also more likely to be nursed to sleep and, thus, to develop negative sleep associations.
- **Achievement of normal developmental milestones,** both motoric milestones (e.g., pulling to stand, crawling) and cognitive development (e.g., separation anxiety), often coincide with an exacerbation or resurgence of nightwakings, especially between the ages of 9 and 12 months.
- **Sleep-disrupting events,** such as illness, vacations, and scheduling changes, can result in disrupted sleep and increased nightwakings.
- **Colic or other medical conditions,** such as otitis media, may result in more frequent nighttime arousals. In addition, in those conditions that typically

require nighttime parental intervention (such as colic), it may be difficult for parents to differentiate between nightwakings due to ongoing physical symptoms and those related to learned behaviors (parental attention to crying).

Other risk factors for problematic nightwakings include:

- **Difficult temperament,** which has been noted to be related to sleep difficulties, especially nightwakings, likely due to the child's inability to self-soothe.
- **Insecure maternal–child attachment,** as infants who are insecurely attached are reported to have more sleep problems, although sleep problems do not necessarily imply that there should be concerns about attachment.
- **Parental anxiety,** especially common in first-time parents, as these parents are more likely to respond immediately to their baby throughout the night, often interfering with the child's returning to sleep independently. In addition, negative emotional states and heightened arousal in parents are likely to increase the arousal level in the infant as well, making settling more difficult.
- **Maternal depression** has also been linked to children's sleep problems. Infant and toddler sleep disturbances clearly contribute to maternal depression, but longitudinal studies indicate an increased risk of sleep disturbances in children of mothers who have previously been identified as depressed.

PRESENTATION/SYMPTOMS

- **Nightwakings**, which require parental intervention for the child to return to sleep. It should be noted that research, clinical, and individual parental definitions of "problematic" nightwakings in terms of frequency, length, and chronicity of the wakings may differ substantially. In clinical practice, however, it is the parents' definition of a "problem" that warrants further assessment and possibly intervention.

Diagnostic Criteria

See Table 7.1.

Associated Features

- **Difficulties at naptime**, also related to the development of negative sleep associations.
- **Delayed sleep onset,** as the transition to sleep may be prolonged if the association requires continued effort, such as a parent continuously rubbing the child's back or a child sucking on a pacifier without letting it fall out of the mouth. Furthermore, many parents who rock or hold their child to sleep find it difficult to make the transition to putting the child down asleep in the crib without waking the child and, thus, needing to start the pattern again.

TABLE 7.1. *Diagnostic criteria: sleep-onset association disorder (307.42)*

A. The patient has a complaint of insomnia.
B. The complaint is temporarily associated with absence of certain conditions (e.g., being held, rocked, or nursed at the breast; listening to the radio; or watching television).
C. The disorder has been present for at least 3 weeks.
D. With the particular association present, sleep is normal in onset, duration, and quality.
E. Polysomnographic monitoring demonstrates:
    1. Normal timing, duration, and quality of the sleep period when the associations are present.
    2. Sleep latency and the duration or number of awakenings can be increased when the associations are absent.
F. No significant underlying mental or medical disorder accounts for the complaint.
G. The symptoms do not meet the criteria for any other sleep disorder causing difficulty initiating sleep (e.g., limit-setting sleep disorder).

Minimal criteria: A plus B plus D plus F plus G.
Used with permission from American Academy of Sleep Medicine. *The international classification of sleep disorders, revised: diagnostic and coding manual.* Westchester, IL: AASM, 1997: 97–98.

- **Daytime behavior problems**, such as irritability and an increase in temper tantrums, associated with the sleep deprivation resulting from nighttime awakenings.
- **Family stress**, including parental sleep disruption, psychiatric symptomatology (including postpartum depression), marital discord, and overall family tension, often results from nighttime sleep disturbances. Studies indicate that behavioral interventions not only result in fewer sleep problems for the child, but they may also alleviate parental stress, improve parental sleep, and generalize to improvements in parenting skills and management of daytime behaviors.

Early Risers

There are two groups of young children who awaken "too early" in the morning (usually determined by parental definition of what is considered too early). The first group are those children who have obtained adequate sleep and whose normal waking time is early in the morning ("larks"). The second group are those who awaken before they get enough sleep. These early-morning awakenings are usually a final nighttime awakening and are maintained by a negative sleep association (e.g., nursing, rocking) or poor limit setting (e.g., parent allows child to join him or her in the parent's bed or to watch early-morning television). Because a significant amount of sleep has already been obtained, the child may be up for a prolonged time; however, the child returns to sleep within an hour or so for an early morning nap or is tired and irritable. Once behavioral interventions are instituted, these children begin to sleep until a more appropriate waketime.

EVALUATION

- **Medical history:** Generally benign.
- **Developmental history:** Developmentally delayed children often have sleep problems that reflect the child's developmental (younger) age rather than chronological age.
- **Family history:** May be positive for psychopathology, especially depression.
- **Behavioral assessment:** Children with a difficult temperament are at increased risk for sleep disturbances related to dysregulation.
- **Nightwaking history:** parents often identify sleep associations as the "trick" that gets the child to fall asleep or return to sleep (e.g., nursing, bottle feeding, rocking).
- **Physical examination:** Usually noncontributory.
- **Diagnostic tests:** Not indicated although a pH probe or milk scan may be considered if there is a concern regarding gastroesophageal reflux.

DIFFERENTIAL DIAGNOSIS

The diagnosis of behaviorally based nightwakings is usually straightforward. However, other causes of nighttime awakenings need to be considered:

- **Medical concerns,** including reflux and pain (especially related to otitis media), often result in prolonged nighttime awakenings, delayed return to sleep, and parental inability to console the child. However, continued parental reinforcement of these nightwakings after the medical condition has resolved may contribute to maintaining them.
- **Underlying sleep disrupter,** such as periodic limb movement disorder (see Chapter 14) or obstructive sleep apnea (see Chapter 13), that contributes to increased nighttime arousals and awakenings.
- **Poor limit setting,** which is usually characterized by the parent's failure to set limits during the night (e.g., allowing the child to watch television in the middle of the night) or reinforcement of inappropriate nighttime behaviors (e.g., bringing the child to the parents' bed on a nightly basis).
- **Inadequate sleep** may increase arousals during sleep. Insufficient sleep can be the result of poor napping or premature discontinuation of naps by parents, an inappropriately late bedtime, inadequate time in bed, or the result of another sleep disorder.
- **Transient sleep disturbances** usually occur in a child with previous normal sleep. Transient nightwakings can be the result of a stressful life event, disruption of sleep schedule (e.g., trip, jet lag), or an illness. Short-term sleep disturbances, however, can become chronic if parents respond in a way (reinforcement of the nightwakings) that fosters inappropriate sleep habits.
- **Inadequate sleep hygiene,** including maintaining an erratic sleep schedule, use of caffeine or other substances, and inadequate sleep may contribute to disturbed sleep and nightwakings.

- **Environmental contributors,** such as a bedroom that is not conducive to sleep (e.g., noisy, hot) or disruption of sleep by others (e.g., parent waking in early morning for work) can cause an increase in the number and duration of awakenings.

MANAGEMENT

When to Refer

Children or adolescents with persistent nightwakings that are not responsive to simple behavioral measures or that are extremely disruptive to the family should be referred to a sleep specialist or a professional who specializes in behavior management. If there is a concern about the existence of an underlying sleep disorder or a medical problem, appropriate referral is warranted.

Treatment

Management of nightwakings should include establishment of a set sleep schedule and bedtime routine. In addition, an intervention strategy should be chosen based on the temperament of the child and parental tolerance, as well as the parenting style of the family. Thus, the behavioral intervention should be tailored to the needs and special circumstances of the individual child and family, and have a high likelihood of success. For example, some families are likely to accept and tolerate prolonged crying at bedtime. Other families will require a more moderate approach in which they gradually make changes (e.g., first three nights establish a bedtime routine only, next three nights rock baby to sleep while gradually weaning off bottle).

- **Sleep habits**
  - **Institution of a sleep schedule** that ensures adequate sleep, as sleep deprivation results in increased nighttime arousals. A bedtime should be set that is appropriate for the child's age and that provides adequate sleep at night. A consistent nightly bedtime will also help to set the circadian clock and enable the child to fall asleep more easily.
  - **Establishment of a consistent bedtime routine** that is approximately 20–45 minutes and includes three to four soothing activities (e.g., bath, pajamas, stories).
  - **Maintenance of daytime sleep (naps)** at least through the age of 3 to 3½ years, as sleep deprivation in a young child will *increase* nighttime arousals and thus *increase* sleep problems.
  - **Transitional objects,** such as a blanket, doll, or stuffed animal. One study found that giving a child a knotted T-shirt previously worn by his or mother (so that it has absorbed her scent) can be an effective transitional object.
- **Parents should not respond immediately** to a baby's movements or sounds to allow the baby a chance to return to sleep independently. Often a parent's response will contribute to a prolonged arousal.

"Drowsy But Awake"

The key to a successful transition from relying on parental intervention to self-soothing to fall asleep is to have the child put to bed "drowsy but awake" at bedtime. This will encourage the development of self-soothing skills, which will generalize to self-soothing back to sleep following normal nighttime arousals.

- **Extinction ("crying it out")** involves putting the child to bed at a designated bedtime and then systematically ignoring the child until a set time the next morning. Extinction has been documented to be a successful treatment; however, it is often not an acceptable choice for families. Parents are often concerned about the effects of the treatment on their child's emotional development and are, thus, less likely to be compliant.
- **Graduated extinction** involves putting the child to bed drowsy but awake and waiting progressively longer periods of time, usually in 5-minute increments, before checking on the child. On each subsequent night, the initial waiting period before checking is increased by 5 minutes. Clinical experience indicates that there is no recommended "optimal" period of time between checks, and that the exact amount of time should be determined by the parents' tolerance for crying and the child's temperament (some children become more agitated with brief parental checks, for example). Since the key to this treatment is to allow the child to fall asleep independently and, thus, develop self-soothing skills, parents can choose how frequently or infrequently they check. When parents check on their child, they should reassure the child but keep contact brief (1–2 minutes) and neutral (e.g., pat on shoulder rather than pick up and cuddle). Research has also indicated that graduated extinction is effective even if instituted only at bedtime, as generalization of self-soothing skills to nighttime arousals will typically occur within 1–2 weeks of the child's falling asleep easily and quickly at bedtime. Thus, parents can institute checking at bedtime only, responding to their child in their usual manner throughout the night (e.g., nursing, bringing child to parents' bed). A similar checking routine during the night may need to be instituted several weeks later if nightwakings persist.

  The success of graduated extinction is usually based on the parents' ability to be consistent and follow through. Thus, "proactive problem-solving" with the family, including discussing potential pitfalls (e.g., child becoming so upset that he or she vomits) and anticipation of problems (e.g., waking an older sibling), greatly increases the likelihood of success. Parents should be warned that the second night of intervention is often more difficult than the first night because of the extinction burst (intensification of crying), but they should also be told that they may expect significant improvement in nightwakings generally within 3–7 days.

Sleep Training for Parents

- **Step 1.** Establish a set bedtime and regular sleep schedule.
- **Step 2.** Develop a consistent bedtime routine in which the activities occurring closest to "lights out" occur in the room where your child sleeps. Avoid making bedtime feedings part of the routine after 6 months.
- **Step 3.** Make the bedroom environment the same at bedtime as it is throughout the night (e.g., lights, music).
- **Step 4.** Put your child to bed drowsy but awake.
- **Step 5.** Check on your child on a preestablished schedule that takes into account the child's temperament and your tolerance for crying. The goal is to allow your child to fall asleep independently.
- **Step 6.** Respond to your baby as usual (rocking, soothing) following nighttime awakenings. The self-soothing skills (falling asleep easily and quickly) that the baby develops at bedtime are highly likely to generalize to self-soothing during the night within 2 weeks.

- **Fading of adult intervention** is appropriate for families who are unable to tolerate the above extinction approaches or consider them to be unacceptable. A plan should be developed that gradually fades (eliminates) adult intervention. In order to develop such a strategy, the end goal should be identified (e.g., falling asleep independently at bedtime) and successive steps to achieving that goal specifically outlined (e.g., 3 days of establishing a bedtime routine and setting bedtime; 3 nights of parent sitting with baby while baby falls asleep in crib; 3 nights of parents sitting 3 feet from crib while baby falls asleep; 3 nights of sitting in doorway; 3 nights of sitting outside doorway; and so forth). Similar strategies can be implemented during the night. Again, initially parents can start with instituting treatment at bedtime only and responding to their child in their usual manner throughout the night, as generalization to nightwakings often occurs (although nighttime intervention may be required 2–3 weeks later). However, some parents may decide to respond to their child's nightwakings in the exact same manner as at bedtime (e.g., if sitting 3 feet from crib at bedtime, will sit 3 feet from crib when child awakens) to provide a consistent response at all sleep times.
- **Discontinuation of nighttime feedings** is appropriate in a baby older than 6 months. There is no evidence that night feedings increase the quality or quantity of sleep and in most cases are not physiologically necessary after 6 months of age. If the bedtime transition to sleep onset routinely occurs in the context of bottle feeding (or nursing), night feeding may become a necessary component of the infant's returning to sleep following nightwakings. The need for feedings during the night may also become a learned behavior ("learned

hunger"), which leads to more frequent and prolonged nightwakings. Night-time feedings can be weaned abruptly ("cold turkey approach") or can be decreased gradually by 1 ounce (bottle fed) or 1 minute (breast fed) per night.

- **Reinforcement strategies** (e.g., sticker charts) can be beneficial with preschoolers and older children. In devising such a system, note that it is most effective if rewards are given immediately (e.g., sticker first thing in the morning with an immediate reward) and obtainable goals are established (e.g., sticker may be earned initially just for sleeping in own bed all night, even in the face of frequent calls to parents) to reinforce success. With time, more challenging goals can be implemented (e.g., sticker obtained for sleeping in bed all night without calling to parents), with less frequent rewards (e.g., 5 stickers per week instead of 3 required to obtain a reward).

- **Collaboration with a behavior therapist** in designing and implementing treatment plans may be prudent if there are complex, chronic, or multiple sleep problems, or if initial behavioral strategies have failed.

"Family Bed" versus " Ferber Method"

There is a great deal of public debate by family bed advocates (e.g., Sears) against graduated-extinction approaches (dubbed the "Ferber method" or "cry it out" approaches). Family bed advocates claim that co-sleeping is more natural and promotes attachment. In contrast, allowing a child to "cry it out" at bedtime or during the night will result in psychological damage and will interfere with parent–child attachment and prolonged breast feeding. At this time, there are no research studies that have provided support for better parent-child attachment related to the family bed **or** for negative repercussions of behavioral interventions. In actuality, research has indicated improved attachment and mood in children, as well as improved family well-being, following behavioral treatment.

Overall, there is no correct response to this age-old debate; rather, it is an individually based family decision. The choice will depend on parenting style, parental tolerance, and child temperament.

PROGNOSIS

Studies indicate that nightwakings are likely to persist without intervention, although negative sleep associations that are established during infancy often taper off following the age of 3 or 4 years, when these behaviors markedly decrease (e.g., bottles/pacifiers/nursing, rocking, holding). However, if the child requires parental presence to fall asleep, the sleep disturbance may continue through middle childhood.

Tips for Talking to Parents

- **Explain that the nighttime arousals are part of the normal sleep pattern** and that the nightwakings per se are not problematic. The concern is rather that the child fails to return to sleep independently (has not learned to self-soothe) and, thus, requires parental intervention to go back to sleep.
- **Discuss sleep associations at bedtime** and their role in perpetuating nightwakings.
- **Develop an appropriate sleep schedule** that ensures adequate sleep and avoids sleep deprivation.
- **Discuss developmentally appropriate parental responses** to and strategies for handling nightwakings.
- **Institute sleep training** at bedtime only, with the goal of developing self-soothing skills and more appropriate sleep associations that will likely generalize to nighttime arousals.
- **Refer for behavioral management** if the nightwakings are severe and unresponsive to simple behavioral interventions.

See Appendix F2 for parent handout on nightwakings.

8

Nighttime Fears

Nighttime fears are common, and typically both normal and benign. Most children experience bedtime or middle of the night fears at some point during childhood, and these are usually considered a normal aspect of development. These fears characteristically begin to occur during the preschool years as children develop the cognitive capacity to understand that they can get hurt or be harmed. The types of fears that children typically have vary at different developmental stages; while young children are often afraid of monsters and other imaginary creatures, older children are more likely to fear being harmed or hurt by more realistic dangers, such as burglars or natural disasters.

Nighttime Fears

Nighttime fears are highly prevalent in preschool-aged children, paralleling cognitive development. Fears are usually short-lived and benign, but must be differentiated from pathologic fears, nightmares, and anxiety disorders.

EPIDEMIOLOGY

Studies indicate that almost all children experience nighttime fears, with the prevalence peaking between the ages of 3 and 6 years. There appears to be a second peak in complaints of nighttime fears in latency-aged girls, especially those who are highly anxious during the day.

ETIOLOGY/RISK FACTORS

Anxiety, stress, and traumatic events have been linked to nighttime fears. Parental anxiety and family conflict may also play a role in exacerbating nighttime fears in children by increasing the level of emotional arousal in the child.

> ### Common Fears at Different Ages
>
> - **Infants**: stimuli in the immediate environment (loud noises, sudden moves)
> - **Toddlers**: strangers, separation, lack of physical support, strange places, heights
> - **Preschoolers**: being alone, the dark, imaginary creatures, animals, thunder, bodily injury, blood/needles
> - **School-aged children**: threats to self-esteem, social or testing situations, bodily injury/illness, supernatural phenomenon, natural disasters
> - **Adolescents**: future events, the unknown, performance failure

PRESENTATION/SYMPTOMS

- **Fearful behaviors,** such as crying, clinging, and leaving the bedroom to seek parental reassurance, at bedtime or in the middle of the night.
- **Bedtime resistance,** including refusal to go to bed or requiring a parent to be present at bedtime.
- **"Curtain calls,"** characterized by frequent requests of parents (e.g., drinks, kisses) after lights out.
- **Partial or complete alleviation of fears** in the context of sharing a room with sibling or other household member.

ASSOCIATED FEATURES

- **Daytime fears,** which may involve similar or different fears.
- **Somatic complaints at bedtime,** including headaches and stomachaches.

EVALUATION

- **Medical history:** Generally benign.
- **Developmental history:** Types of fears experienced by developmentally delayed children generally reflect the child's developmental age rather than chronological age.
- **Family history:** Anxiety disorders in the family suggest the potential for more global anxiety problems in the child.
- **Behavioral assessment:** Presence of daytime anxiety symptoms or oppositional behavior may suggest more global behavioral problems. It is also important to elicit a detailed description of the typical parental response to the fearful behavior.
- **Physical examination:** Usually noncontributory.
- **Diagnostic tests:** Not indicated.

DIFFERENTIAL DIAGNOSIS

Diagnosis of nighttime fears is usually straightforward; however, other disorders should be considered:

- **Bedtime resistance.** Some children learn that expressing fears is an effective stalling tactic or a way to avoid bedtime, especially because parents may respond more positively to fearful behaviors than they do to oppositional behavior. These parental responses may then serve to reinforce fearful behaviors. The bedtime resistance, in turn, may be related to any number of different sleep problems, including limit-setting sleep disorder (see Chapter 6) and sleep phase delay (see Chapter 16).
- **Nightmares.** Frightening dreams that awaken a child during the night may contribute to the development of a conditioned fear, as well as avoidance of bedtime and falling asleep (see Chapter 9).
- **Phobias.** Phobias are conditioned, persistent, and often quite dramatic fear responses to specific stimuli (dogs) or circumstances (riding on elevators) that typically occur during the day as well and significantly impact on daytime functioning.
- **Anxiety disorders.** Children and adolescents with anxiety disorders, including generalized anxiety disorder, posttraumatic stress disorder, and separation anxiety disorder, frequently present with nighttime fears. The fearful behavior is usually present concomitantly during the day, and functioning is impacted. In addition, the degree, duration, and pervasiveness of the symptoms help differentiate situational and transient nighttime anxiety from a more chronic and global anxiety disorder.
- **Child abuse.** Children who have experienced physical, sexual, or emotional abuse may have nighttime fears, but these are generally severe and persistent and are accompanied by significant physiologic arousal. Many of these children also have significant daytime symptoms, including anxiety, withdrawal, and depressive symptomatology.

MANAGEMENT

When to Refer

Children or adolescents with persistent or severe bedtime fears that are not responsive to simple behavioral measures should be referred to a mental health professional.

Treatment

An important aspect in counseling parents on how to respond to nighttime fears is to have the parents maintain a balance between reassuring the child and avoiding reinforcement of the fears. If a child or adolescent is reassured too much, the parents may be subtly providing positive attention for the fearful behavior, thus increasing the likelihood that it will reoccur. In addition, some children may interpret their parents' concern about the fears as tacit proof that the fears are well founded. In general, strategies aimed at younger children more often involve parental reassurance while older children typically benefit from an approach that includes teaching and positive reinforcement for independent coping skills.

Suggestions for ways parents can respond to their child's nighttime fears:

- **Reassure and communicate the idea of safety,** such as having parents repeatedly tell the child that he or she is safe and that the parents are always nearby and will make sure that nothing bad happens (e.g., "Mommy and Daddy are right downstairs and we'll always make sure that you are safe.").
- **Teach the child developmentally appropriate coping skills** and discuss alternative ways to respond to nighttime fears, such as "being brave" and making positive self-statements (e.g., "Monsters are just pretend."). Another strategy is to provide examples of coping role models by reading stories about children who are afraid and conquer their fears.
- **Develop creative solutions,** such as the use of "monster spray" (parent fills a spray bottle with water and sprays the child's room and closet at bedtime), although it should be noted that some young children may view this as evidence that a monster actually exists! Having a pet as a nighttime companion or having siblings share a bedroom are alternative strategies that work for some families. Whenever possible, the child should be actively involved in generating solutions to foster a sense of mastery and control.
- **Encourage the use of security objects,** as they can be comforting to the child.
- **Use a nightlight** to decrease a child's fear of the dark or monsters.
- **Leave the bedroom door open,** so that a child does not feel isolated.
- **Avoid television shows and movies** that may be frightening or overstimulating, particularly just before bedtime.
- **Teach the child relaxation strategies,** such as deep breathing or visual imagery (e.g., imagining a beach or other favorite scene), which can help a child relax at bedtime and fall asleep more easily.
- **Discuss the child's fears** and alternative ways to respond to the fears during the day rather than in the evening, as this is less likely to provoke anxiety.
- **Set appropriate, firm, and consistent limits** on bedtime behavior to avoid reinforcing the child's "being scared." For example, a parent might say, "Remember, no crying and no calling at bedtime."
- **Institute a "checking system" at bedtime** to provide the child with a predictable schedule (e.g., every 10 minutes) of parental reassurance. This has the benefit of making parental contact noncontingent on the child's behavior (e.g., calling out).
- **Encourage the child to remain in bed or in the bedroom,** so that he or she does not become conditioned to avoid the bedroom. If parental presence is

temporarily required to alleviate the child's fears, it is generally better for parents to stay in the child's room rather than to have the child join the parents in their room.

• **Develop a reward system for appropriate bedtime behavior** (stickers for being a "big boy") rather than reinforcing (with attention) the learned fearful behavior (e.g., "I'm scared."). Appropriate behaviors that are required for positive reinforcement should be as specific as possible (staying in bed all night, not calling out after lights out), and the reward schedule should be set up to offer a high likelihood of the child's being successful (e.g., nightly reward).

PROGNOSIS

Nighttime fears that are part of normal developmental are usually short-lived and disappear by age 5 or 6. Fears may become more chronic in a child or adolescent with an anxiety disorder.

Tips for Talking to Parents

• **Distinguish between normal and pathologic fears.**
• **Explain that normal nighttime fears are part of normal cognitive development.**
• **Discuss treatment options and parents' response to fearful behavior.**
• **Reinforce establishment of appropriate sleep habits and parental limit-setting.**

See Appendix F3 for parent handout on nighttime fears.

9

Nightmares

Nightmares are frightening dreams that usually awaken a child or adolescent, leaving the child upset and in need of comfort. Although some individuals distinguish between nightmares, which awaken the sleeper, and bad dreams, which do not, this distinction is somewhat arbitrary. When the nightmare involves awakening, most children are afraid to return to sleep and seek comfort. Given that very young children often cannot distinguish between a dream and reality, they may insist that something fearful continues to exist.

Nightmares

Nightmares are frightening dreams, occurring during REM sleep, that usually result in an awakening from sleep.

The content of nightmares usually differs across the ages and reflects common developmental issues. Most young toddlers have concerns about being separated from their parents. By age 2 years, nightmares begin to incorporate monsters and other frightening imaginary creatures. For young children, nightmares may also involve a recent traumatic event (e.g., getting lost, being immunized, being barked at by a large dog). Older children often have nightmares related to frightening or upsetting movies, television programs, stories, or a disturbing daytime experience. Nightmares may also coincide with a stressor or traumatic event (e.g., being away overnight, starting a new school).

EPIDEMIOLOGY

Studies indicate that approximately 75% of children report experiencing at least one nightmare, and 10% to 50% of young children have nightmares that result in parental interaction during the night. One study reported prevalence rates for chronic nightmares, defined as a nightmare problem lasting longer than 3 months, as 24% for ages 2 to 5 years and 41% for ages 6 to 10 years.

ETIOLOGY/RISK FACTORS

- **Stress and/or traumatic events,** including child abuse.
- **Anxiety and anxiety disorders,** which can lead to both increased frequency and severity of nightmares.
- **Sleep deprivation,** which can result in intense and vivid dreams due to increased rebound REM sleep.
- **Medications** that have a direct effect on the amount (increased) of REM sleep, or are REM suppressants whose withdrawal leads to REM rebound (see Chapter 19).

PRESENTATION/SYMPTOMS

Children or adolescents with nightmares will usually recall at least fragmented and often detailed scary dream content and will awaken frightened but coherent. In addition, if awakening occurs, the child or adolescent is often afraid to return to sleep and will seek parental reassurance.

Diagnostic Criteria

See Table 9.1.

Associated Features

- **Daytime fears.** Many children with nightmares also report nighttime fears (see Chapter 8).
- **Bedtime resistance.** Some children develop a conditioned aversion to their bed or bedtime because they associate sleep with nightmares.

TABLE 9.1. *Diagnostic criteria: nightmares (307.47)*

A. The patient has at least one episode of sudden awakening from sleep with intense fear, anxiety, and feeling of impending harm.
B. The patient has immediate recall of frightening dream content.
C. Full alertness occurs immediately upon awakening, with little confusion or disorientation.
D. Associated features include at least one of the following:
    1. Return to sleep after the episode is delayed and not rapid
    2. The episode occurs during the latter half of the habitual sleep period
E. Polysomnographic monitoring demonstrates the following:
    1. An abrupt awakening from at least 10 minutes of REM sleep
    2. Mild tachycardia and tachypnea during the episode
    3. Absence of epileptic activity in association with the disorder
F. Other sleep disorders, such as sleep terrors and sleep walking, can occur.

Minimal criteria: A plus B plus C plus D.
Used with permission from American Academy of Sleep Medicine. *The international classification of sleep disorders, revised: diagnostic and coding manual.* Westchester, IL: AASM, 1997:165.

EVALUATION

- **Nightmare history:** In evaluating nightmares, both chronicity and severity should be carefully assessed, as nightmare severity is more likely to be related to psychopathology.
- **Medical history:** Generally benign.
- **Developmental history:** Developmentally delayed children may be less able to verbalize concerns about nightmares.
- **Family history:** The ubiquitous nature of nightmares in the general population makes a positive family history nonspecific. However, parents who have experienced frequent or troublesome frightening dreams may respond differently to their child's nightmares (e.g., more attention, anxiety).
- **Behavioral assessment:** A history of more global anxiety, regression in behavior, or extreme arousal in association with nightmares should raise concerns about the possibility of abuse or trauma.
- **Physical examination:** Usually noncontributory.
- **Diagnostic tests:**
  - **A sleep diary** that documents the frequency of nightmares over a period of several weeks and the duration of associated nightwakings may be helpful.

DIFFERENTIAL DIAGNOSIS

- **Sleep terrors.** Parents often have a difficult time distinguishing between nightmares and sleep terrors. Nightmares, in comparison to sleep terrors (see chart in Chapter 10), usually have the following features:
  - Occurrence in the latter half of the night, when REM sleep predominates
  - Recollection of dream content
  - Total recall for the event
  - No confusion or disorientation
  - Delayed return to sleep
- **Psychiatric disorder.** Frequent nightmares may be associated with a psychiatric disorder, including anxiety disorders, bipolar disorder, and schizophrenia.

MANAGEMENT

When to Refer

Children or adolescents with persistent or severe nightmares that are not responsive to simple behavioral measures or that are extremely disruptive should be referred to a mental health professional for evaluation and treatment.

Treatment

In general, as with other anxiety-associated behavioral issues, strategies for dealing with nightmares aimed at younger children more often involve active parental reassurance, whereas older children may benefit more from an approach that includes teaching and positive reinforcement for independent coping skills.

Suggestions for ways parents can manage their child's nightmares:

Reduce the likelihood of nightmares:
- **Avoid exposure to frightening or overstimulating images,** especially just before bedtime, including frightening stories, movies, and television shows.
- **Reduce stressors,** as persistent nightmares may indicate stress or an ongoing concern.
- **Ensure adequate sleep,** as sleep deprivation contributes to increased nightmare frequency.
- **Parental response to nightmares:**
  - **Reassurance by parents** that "it was only a dream." It is important that parents remain calm and matter of fact, and strike a balance between reassuring the child and not providing excessive attention. If the child gets out of bed, the parent should calmly escort the child back to bed and briefly provide reassurance there. Further discussion of the nightmare should be postponed until the following day, when alternative coping strategies for the future may be discussed.
  - **Security objects** can be comforting and facilitate a faster return to sleep. Some children find the presence of a family pet reassuring.
  - **Dim, low-level nightlight** can be helpful.
  - **Encouragement of verbal children to use their imagination** may help alleviate nightmares. Effective strategies may include drawing a picture that represents the bad dreams and then crumpling it up and throwing it away, devising a positive ending to the dream, or hanging a dream catcher over the bed.

Additional treatment strategies:
- **Relaxation strategies,** including progressive muscle relaxation (PMR) and guided imagery. Relaxation tapes can be obtained through the Anxiety Disorder Association of America (ADAA; *www.adaa.org*) or the Child Anxiety Network (*www.childanxiety.net*).
- **Systematic desensitization,** combined with relaxation strategies, which can be used to countercondition the anxiety response. Systematic desensitization involves developing a hierarchy of fear-invoking activities or thoughts from least to most frightening with the child (e.g., looking at a picture of a dog, watching a friend play with a puppy, petting a large dog). These activities or thoughts are paired with a relaxing activity (deep breathing, progressive muscle relaxation) that counters the fear response. This technique may be particularly helpful with nightmares that have a recurrent specific theme.
- **See Chapter 8** for additional treatment strategies.

PROGNOSIS

Nightmares are usually short lived but may persist in some children or adolescents, especially if the nightmares are related to a traumatic event.

Tips for Talking to Parents

- **Explain that nightmares** are virtually universal and are part of normal cognitive development, usually peaking between 3 and 6 years of age.
- **Discuss developmentally appropriate parental responses** to and strategies for handling nightmares.
- **Develop an appropriate sleep schedule** that ensures adequate sleep and avoids sleep deprivation.
- **Discuss any recent stressors or traumatic events that may be contributory,** while reassuring parents that the vast majority of the time nightmares are isolated events.
- **Refer for psychological evaluation** if the nightmares are highly persistent or severe and unresponsive to simple behavioral interventions.

See Appendix F4 for parent handout on nightmares.

10

Sleepwalking and Sleep Terrors

Sleepwalking (somnambulism) and **sleep terrors** (pavor nocturnus), often referred to as **partial arousal parasomnias,** are episodic sleep disorders that share a common underlying pathophysiology and have a number of overlapping clinical features. The partial arousal parasomnias share characteristics of both the waking and deep sleep states, and involve autonomic or skeletal muscle disturbances, autonomic behaviors, and disorientation. Sleepwalking and sleep terrors occur almost exclusively during slow-wave sleep (stages 3 and 4 of non-REM sleep) and therefore do not involve dreaming. These two disorders usually occur within 1 to 2 hours after sleep onset, last from a few minutes to an hour, and are characterized by retrograde amnesia. During an episode, children or adolescents have the appearance of being awake, and most children avoid comfort or soothing, which may be disturbing to parents. Although they may be triggered by stress, neither behavior indicates a primary underlying psychological problem or trauma.

Common Characteristics of Partial Arousal Parasomnias

- Occurrence within the first few hours of the night
- Agitation and confusion
- Avoidance of comfort
- Retrograde amnesia
- Exacerbation of sleep deprivation or an underlying sleep disrupter

---

Sleepwalking is a common and benign sleep behavior. During sleepwalking, the eyes are usually open, the child may appear confused or dazed, and he or she may mumble or give inappropriate answers to questions. Occasionally, a sleepwalking child may appear agitated. A sleepwalker is often clumsy and may perform bizarre or strange actions, such as urinating in a closet. Sleepwalking can occur infrequently or on a nightly basis.

Sleepwalking

Sleepwalking is a benign and common behavior in children, occurring during the first few hours of the night when slow-wave sleep (stages 3 and 4 of non-REM sleep) is predominant.

Sleep terrors, or night terrors, are dramatic events and, as such, can be distressing to parents or caregivers (these episodes are referred to as sleep terrors rather than night terrors because they can occur during any sleep period, including naps). As disturbing and frightening as these events appear to the observer, the child is totally unaware of his or her behavior. Paradoxically, sleep terrors are much worse to watch than to experience, and much less traumatic to the child than a nightmare or bad dream.

Sleep Terrors

Sleep terrors are characterized by a sudden arousal from slow-wave sleep, accompanied by autonomic and behavioral manifestations of intense fear.

EPIDEMIOLOGY

- **Sleepwalking.** Between 15% and 40% of children sleepwalk on at least one occasion, with 3% to 4% having frequent (weekly, monthly) episodes. Onset of episodes is usually between 4 and 6 years, and peak occurrence is between 4 and 8 years. About one-third of sleepwalkers have episodes over a 5-year span; about 10% will continue to sleep walk for 10 years.
- **Sleep terrors.** Approximately 3% of children experience sleep terrors, primarily during the preschool and elementary school years, and the age of onset is usually between 4 and 12 years. The frequency of episodes is often highest at the onset and tends to be higher with younger age of onset. Because of the common genetic predisposition, the prevalence of sleep terrors in children who sleepwalk is about 10%. Although sleep terrors can occur at any age from infancy through adulthood, most individuals outgrow sleep terrors by adolescence.

ETIOLOGY/RISK FACTORS

- **Positive family history.** There is frequently a genetic component in partial arousal parasomnias, with an 80% to 90% likelihood that a child with sleepwalking or sleep terrors has an affected first-degree relative.

- **Other associated conditions.** Partial arousal parasomnias appear to be more common in individuals with migraine headaches and Tourette syndrome, possibly related to alterations in serotonin metabolism.
- **Factors that exacerbate parasomnias.** Partial arousal parasomnias occur almost exclusively in slow-wave sleep. Sleep deprivation/disruption often results in a rebound compensatory increase in slow-wave sleep. Therefore, in general, any condition that disrupts sleep or reduces sleep duration tends to increase the likelihood that a partial arousal parasomnia episode will occur in a susceptible individual. Environmental conditions (e.g., noise) that increase arousals, especially during slow-wave sleep, may also trigger events. Some conditions may also increase the likelihood of partial arousal episodes by decreasing the arousal threshold.

  Exacerbating/trigger factors include:
  - Sleep deprivation (acute or chronic)
  - Irregular sleep schedule
  - Fever and illness
  - Medications (e.g., chloral hydrate)
  - Sleeping with a full bladder
  - Sleeping in a different environment
  - Sleeping in a noisy environment
  - Stress and anxiety

PRESENTATION

Partial arousal parasomnias usually occur in the first few hours after sleep onset and last a few minutes to a half-hour. Frequency ranges from a one-time event to a nightly occurrence; some children may have multiple episodes in a single night.

- **Sleepwalking.** Parents are generally able to identify an event as sleepwalking; occasionally, the presenting complaint is nocturnal episodes that involve unusual or bizarre behaviors (going to a sibling's room in the middle of the night, wandering around downstairs), confusion, agitation, and incoherent responses to questions. Parents are not always able to tell whether their child is awake or asleep at the time.

Injury Risk

Sleepwalking and sleep terrors can lead to physical harm, resulting from falling down stairs, walking into traffic, or trying to escape. Ensurance of safety should be one of the primary concerns of health care practitioners when dealing with partial arousal parasomnias.

- **Sleep terrors.** Sleep terrors usually have a sudden onset, and the child's appearance during one of these episodes is that of extreme agitation, fright, and confusion, often involving crying and/or screaming. Extreme physiologic arousal (e.g., hyperventilation, tachycardia, diaphoresis, dilated pupils) is common. However, sleep terrors may be much milder (sometimes described as a confusional arousal), with the child simply appearing agitated. A child having a sleep terror is often clumsy and may flail, push a parent away, or behave in other strange ways. Because of the dramatic nature of these episodes, parents may be concerned that their child has experienced some emotional or physical trauma; alternatively, parents may also assume that the events themselves result in psychological damage to the child.

Associated Features

- **Impact on social functioning.** Because of the potential embarrassment and the high likelihood of harm, many children and adolescents with parasomnias avoid social situations such as overnight visits to friends or summer camp.
- **Parental anxiety.** Because of the unusual nature of these events, parents are often highly anxious about whether there is an underlying meaning to the episodes, as well as how to respond to the events, and are often concerned about not being present during an event (e.g., avoid use of babysitters, discourage sleepovers).

Diagnostic Criteria

See Tables 10.1 and 10.2.

TABLE 10.1. *Diagnostic criteria: sleepwalking (307.46-0)*

A. The patient exhibits ambulation that occurs in sleep.
B. The onset typically occurs in prepubertal children.
C. Associated features include:
   1. Difficulty in arousing the patient during an episode
   2. Amnesia following an episode
D. Episodes typically occur in the first third of the sleep episode.
E. Polysomnographic monitoring demonstrates the onset of an episode during stage 3 or stage 4 sleep.
F. Other medical and psychiatric disorders can be present but do not account for the symptom.
G. The ambulation is not due to other sleep disorders, such as REM sleep behavior disorder or sleep terrors.

Minimal criteria: A plus B plus C.
Used with permission from American Academy of Sleep Medicine. *The international classification of sleep disorders; revised: diagnostic coding and manual.* Westchester, IL: AASM, 1997:147.

TABLE 10.2. *Diagnostic criteria: sleep terrors (307.46-1)*

A. The patient complains of a sudden episode of intense terror during sleep.
B. The episodes usually occur within the first third of the night.
C. Partial or total amnesia occurs for the events during the episode.
D. Polysomnographic monitoring demonstrates the onset of episodes during stage 3 or stage 4 sleep. Tachycardia usually occurs in association with the episodes.
E. Other medical disorders (e.g., epilepsy) are not the cause of the episode.
F. Other sleep disorders (e.g., nightmares) can be present.

Minimal criteria: A plus B plus C.
Used with permission from American Academy of Sleep Medicine. *The international classification of sleep disorders, revised: diagnostic and coding manual.* Westchester, IL: AASM, 1997:149.

EVALUATION

- **Medical history:** Generally benign. However, history may reveal evidence suggestive of a sleep disorder that results in disrupted and/or insufficient sleep. These include:
  - **Sleep disordered breathing:** An apneic event/arousal can directly trigger an episode, or may increase the likelihood of events by causing sleep disruption and a rebound increase in slow-wave sleep.
  - **Restless legs syndrome and/or periodic limb movement disorder:** Associated sleep deprivation/disruption may increase slow-wave sleep (see Chapter 14).
  - **Behaviorally-based sleep issues:** Frequent nightwakings and prolonged bedtime refusal can result in sleep deprivation, exacerbating parasomnias (see Chapters 6 and 7).
  - **Seizures:** The medical history may also suggest the need to rule out a seizure disorder. Possible risk factors include a history of seizures, as well as unusual characteristics of the episodes themselves such as stereotypic features, multiple nightly occurrences, and late onset (adolescence).
- **Developmental/school history:** Usually normal.
- **Family history:** Often positive for sleepwalking/sleep terrors.
- **Behavioral assessment:** Most children do not have significant behavioral concerns. Because individuals with partial arousal parasomnias are actually asleep during the episodes, sleep disruption and associated evidence of daytime sleepiness are unusual.
- **Physical examination:** Generally unremarkable.
- **Diagnostic tests**
  - **Overnight polysomnography** is not a routine part of the evaluation for partial arousal parasomnias. Because these are episodic events, they may not be captured on a single-night study. However, if there is a concern about another underlying sleep disrupter (e.g., sleep disordered breathing, periodic limb movement disorder), an overnight sleep study may be appropriate. Polysomnography may also be warranted to differentiate between a parasomnia and a seizure disorder (note that only some sleep centers have the capability of a full seizure montage) (Fig. 10.1).

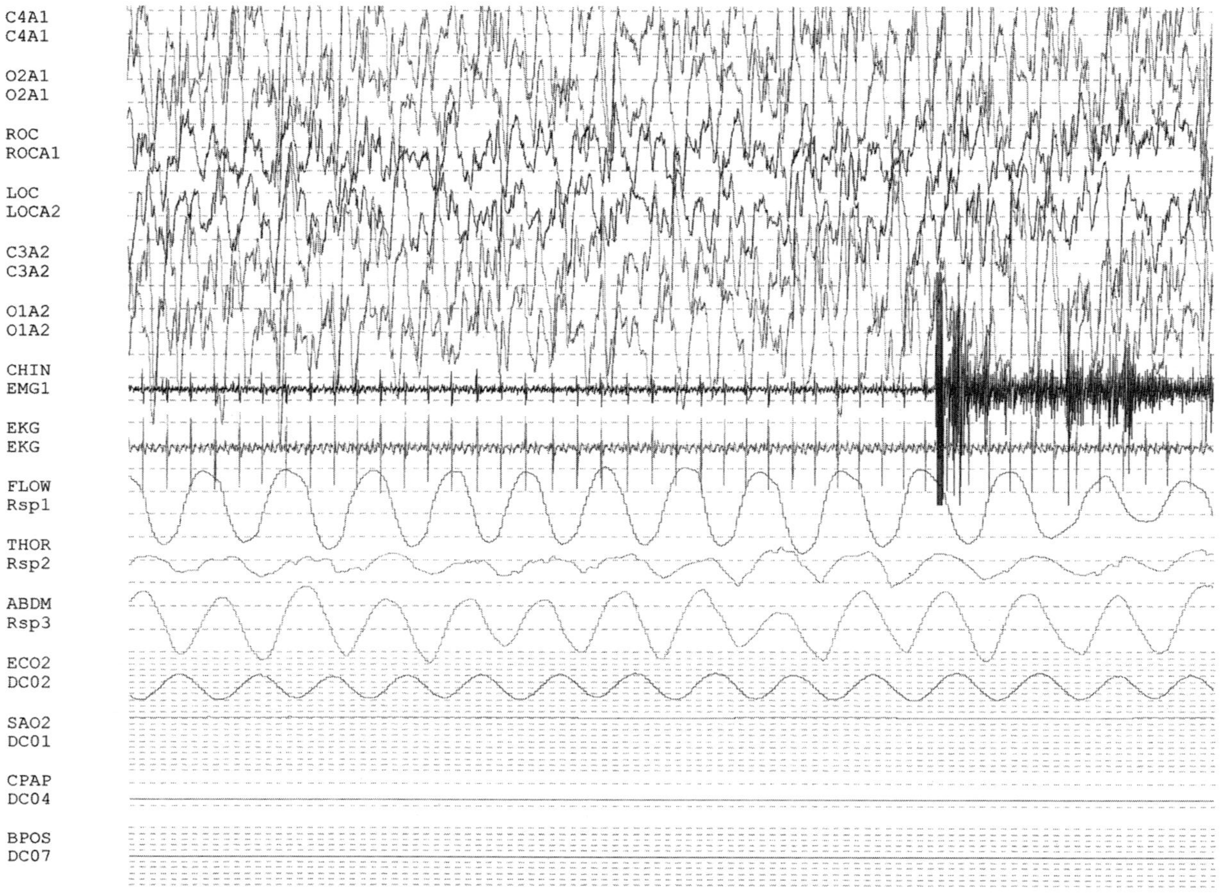

C4A1
C4A1

O2A1
O2A1

ROC
ROCA1

LOC
LOCA2

C3A2
C3A2

O1A2
O1A2

CHIN
EMG1

EKG
EKG

FLOW
Rsp1

THOR
Rsp2

ABDM
Rsp3

ECO2
DCO2

SAO2
DC01

CPAP
DC04

BPOS
DC07

FIG. 10.1. Partial arousal parasomnia.

- **Videotaping** by the parents in the home can help distinguish parasomnias from other behaviors, especially stereotypic behaviors associated with seizures.
- **Sleep diaries** can help the assessment for contributing factors, such as sleep deprivation and irregular sleep schedules.

DIFFERENTIAL DIAGNOSIS

- **Sleep terror versus nightmare versus seizure disorder** (see Table 10.3).
- **Nocturnal panic attacks.** Patient typically has similar episodes that occur in the daytime, and there is recall of the episode the next morning.

MANAGEMENT

When To Refer

Children or adolescents with parasomnias who also present with symptoms of another underlying sleep disrupter (e.g., sleep disordered breathing) should be referred to a sleep specialist. If pharmacologic treatment is being considered, it is also best to consult with a pediatric sleep specialist. Where there are concerns

TABLE 10.3. *Differentiation of episodic nocturnal phenomenon*

Characteristics	Sleepwalking	Sleep terrors	Nightmares	Nocturnal seizures
Timing during night	First third	First third	Last third	Variable; often at sleep-wake transition
Sleep stage	SWS	SWS	REM	Non-REM > REM
Clinical description				
• Displacement from bed	Usual during event	Unusual during event	Occasional after event	Unusual
• Autonomic arousal/ agitation	Low to mild	High to extreme	Mild to high	Variable
• Stereotypic/ repetitive behavior	Variable; complex behaviors	Variable	None; little motor behavior	Common
• Arousal threshold	High; agitated if awakened	High; agitated if awakened	Low; awake and agitated after event	High; awake and confused after event
• Associated daytime sleepiness	None	None	Yes, if night waking prolonged	Probable
Recall of event	None or fragmentary	None or fragmentary	Frequent, vivid	None
Prevalence	Common (20% at least one episode; 1%–6% chronic)	Rare (1%–6%); 10% of sleepwalkers	Very common	Rare
Family history	Common	Common	No	Variable

REM, rapid eye movement; SWS, slow-wave sleep.

regarding stress or other psychological issues, a referral to a mental health specialist is warranted.

Treatment

Management of partial arousal parasomnias should first include **reassurance and education** of the child and family regarding the benign and self-limited nature of the disorder. Parents may be told that most children stop having sleepwalking episodes or sleep terrors by adolescence. Interim management should include institution of appropriate safety measures and discussion of trigger/exacerbating factors. Sleep hygiene and behavioral management of the episodes should be reviewed. However, the decision about whether to actively treat the parasomnias is based on the frequency and severity of the episodes and can involve medication management or scheduled awakenings.

Safety
- **Safety measures,** including use of gates (doorways, top of staircases); locking of outside doors and windows; lighting of hallways; and ensuring the safety of the sleeping environment (e.g., clutter on floors).
- **Parent notification measures,** such as alarm systems or a bell attached to the bedroom door.

Sleep hygiene (e.g., ensure adequate sleep, maintain regular sleep-wake schedule)

Behavioral management
- **Address behaviorally-based nightwakings or bedtime refusal,** which may be contributing to sleep deprivation.
- **Avoid awakening** as attempts to awaken a child during a parasomnia will typical increase agitation and prolong the event.
- **Guide the child back to bed** to encourage return to normal sleep.
- **Avoid interfering** as this can prolong the event. The normal response of parents is to try and comfort their child during one of these episodes, which may increase agitation.
- **Avoid next-day discussions,** as this is likely to worry the child and may lead to bedtime resistance.

Additional treatment
- **Pharmacologic treatment** may be indicated in cases of frequent or severe episodes, high risk of injury, violent behavior, or serious disruption to the family. The primary pharmacologic agents used are short-acting benzodiazepines given as a small dose at bedtime [e.g., clonazepam (Klonopin), 0.25 to 2 mg or oxazepam (Serax), 5 to 20 mg], for 3 to 6 months (until episodes are totally suppressed). Benzodiazepines suppress slow-wave sleep in the first third of the night, thus reducing the likelihood that an episode will occur. Intermittent drug therapy has also been used in patients who have a pattern of events that occur in clusters of days or weeks separated by parasomnia-free periods.

Abrupt discontinuation may result in rebound increased slow-wave sleep, so it is best to taper medication slowly over several weeks. Tricyclic antidepressants (clomipramine, desipramine, imipramine) at bedtime have also been used in patients who are nonresponsive to benzodiazepines.

- **Scheduled awakenings** is a behavioral technique that is most likely to be successful in situations in which partial arousal episodes occur on a nightly basis. Studies have indicated that in children with frequent parasomnias that occur at a highly predictive time scheduled awakenings can be highly effective. Scheduled awakenings involve having the parent wake the child approximately 15 to 30 minutes prior to the time of night that the first parasomnia episode typically occurs. Thus, parents first need to keep a sleep diary that includes the exact time of each episode. The parent then begins awakening the child on a nightly basis, approximately 30 minutes before a usual event, just to the point of arousal (e.g., child changes position or mumbles). For example, if the child usually falls asleep at 8:30 PM and sleepwalks at 10:00 PM, then the parent should institute scheduled awakenings at 9:30 PM. These nightly awakening should be continued for 2 to 4 weeks. If the parasomnias reoccur following discontinuation of the scheduled awakenings, they may be reinstituted for several weeks.

PROGNOSIS

Most children naturally stop sleepwalking or experiencing sleep terrors in childhood. By age 8 years, 50% of children with sleepwalking/terrors no longer experience parasomnias, and most cases resolve spontaneously following puberty as a result of the dramatic decrease in slow-wave sleep.

Tips for Talking to Parents

- **Explain that sleepwalking and sleep terrors are a neurodevelopmental phenomenon.** They are neither indicative of a psychological issue nor result in psychological harm.
- **Ensure safety measures**, including locking of all outside doors and windows.
- **Suggest an appropriate sleep schedule** to ensure adequate sleep.
- **Discourage parental intervention during an episode** as this is likely to increase agitation and prolong the event.
- **Discuss trigger/exacerbating factors**, including sleep deprivation, sleeping in an unfamiliar environment, and illness.
- **Discuss the risks and benefits of treatment options**, including medications and scheduled awakenings in more problematic cases.

See Appendix F5 for parent handout on sleepwalking and F6 on sleep terrors.

11

Headbanging and Bodyrocking

Headbanging (jactatio capitis nocturna) and **bodyrocking** fall under the diagnostic category of rhythmic movement disorders. Rhythmic movement disorders involve repetitive and stereotypic movements of large muscles and occur primarily during sleep–wake transitions; thus, these behaviors may occur not only during sleep onset at bedtime but at naptimes and following nighttime arousals as well. Bodyrocking, headbanging, and bodyrolling are the most common types of rhythmic movements. Children engage in these behaviors as a means of soothing themselves to sleep; rhythmic humming or chanting may accompany the movements. The duration of these behaviors can be from minutes to several hours. Although sometimes distressing to caretakers, significant injury is rare.

In almost all cases, rhythmic movement behaviors are benign and occur in normally developing children. However, in situations that involve children with psychiatric or neurologic disorders, such as developmental delays, autism, or blindness, there may be a risk of potential injury due to the intensity and frequency of the behaviors. These children are much more likely to also engage in these behaviors while awake.

Rhythmic Movement Disorder

Rhythmic movements, including headbanding and bodyrocking, are common in young children and serve as self-soothing behaviors. They can occur both at sleep onset and following normal nighttime arousals.

EPIDEMIOLOGY

- **Prevalence/age of onset.** Studies indicate that approximately two-thirds of 9-month-old infants engage in some type of rhythmic behavior, with less than half continuing these behaviors at 18 months, and only 8% at 4 years of age. It is estimated that 3% to 15% of children have significant headbanging. Most

children who engage in these behaviors have an onset prior to one year of age, with bodyrocking starting at an earlier age than headbanging.
- **Gender.** More common in boys (4:1 ratio).

ETIOLOGY/RISK FACTORS

- **Vestibular stimulation.** An increased need for kinesthetic stimulation may be related to rhythmic behaviors.
- **Nighttime arousals.** Any factor that increases nighttime arousals/awakenings, such as sleep disordered breathing, pain, or gastroesophageal reflux, may provide increased opportunities for the behavior to occur.
- **Parental attention.** Caregivers can reinforce rhythmic behaviors by inadvertently providing attention.
- **Developmental disabilities.** The majority of children who engage in rhythmic behaviors are otherwise normal and healthy. However, rhythmic movement disorder, especially when persistent or also occurring during the day, can be associated with mental retardation, pervasive developmental disorders (including autism), and psychopathology.
- **Additional factors.** Other associated conditions include environmental stress, lack of environmental stimulation, and self-stimulation.

PRESENTATION

Children and adolescents with rhythmic movement disorder typically present with one of the following:

- **Bodyrocking** presents as rocking forward and back, without headbanging, usually while on the hands and knees. Bodyrocking usually begins earliest, at about 6 months of age.
- **Headbanging,** starting around 9 months, can occur in multiple forms:
  - Lying prone and lifting the head to bang down into a pillow or the mattress.
  - Rocking on hands or knees and banging head into the headboard or wall.
  - Sitting upright and banging head back into the headboard or wall.
- **Headrolling** involves side-to-side movements of the head, usually in the supine position, with an average age of onset of 10 months.
- **Bodyrolling** is less common than the other behaviors, and involves rolling of the entire body in a lateral manner (side to side).

Associated Features

- **Disruption to parental sleep** and other family members. This may occur if the rhythmic behavior is loud and occurs both at bedtime and throughout the night.
- **Parental anxiety** as parents are frequently concerned about the risk of injury, especially head trauma. They may also associate these behaviors with mental

TABLE 11.1. Diagnostic criteria: rhythmic movement disorder (307.3)

A. The patient exhibits rhythmic body movements during drowsiness or sleep.
B. At least one of the following types of disorders is present:
  1. The head is forcibly moved in an anterior–posterior direction (headbanging type).
  2. The head is moved laterally while in a supine position (headrolling type).
  3. The whole body is rocked while on the hands and knees (bodyrocking type).
  4. The whole body is moved laterally while in a supine position (bodyrolling type).
C. Onset typically occurs within the first 2 years of life.
D. Polysomnographic monitoring during an episode demonstrates both of the following findings:
  1. Rhythmic movements during any stage of sleep or in wakefulness.
  2. No other seizure activity occurs in association with the disorder.
E. No other medical or mental disorder (e.g., epilepsy) causes the symptom.
F. The symptoms do not meet the diagnostic criteria for other sleep disorders producing abnormal movements during sleep (e.g., sleep bruxism).

Minimal criteria: A plus B.
Used with permission from American Academy of Sleep Medicine. *The international classification of sleep disorders, revised: diagnostic and coding manual.* Westchester, IL: AASM, 1997:154.

retardation and/or autism, and, thus, may have concerns about their child's development.

Diagnostic Criteria

See Table 11.1.

EVALUATION

- **Medical history:** Generally unremarkable. The history should include a complete review for additional factors that may result in increased arousals, including sleep disordered breathing, reflux, and pain related to such factors as an ear infection or headaches.
- **Developmental history:** Usually normal. However, further evaluation for developmental delays in a child with persistent rhythmic behaviors, especially if they also occur during the day, may be warranted. Because sensory deprivation can contribute to the etiology of rhythmic movement disorders, in severe or persistent cases the possibility of child neglect or abuse should be considered.
- **Family history:** May be positive, as there appears to be a genetic component.
- **Behavioral assessment:** Usually does not indicate the existence of behavioral problems, but parental response to the behavior (reinforcement) should be explored. Children who have other self-stimulatory behaviors (e.g., rumination) may be more likely to have experienced neglect.
- **Physical examination:** Usually unremarkable. Occasionally, children may have minor contusions or calluses at the point of impact, but serious injury is rare.

DIFFERENTIAL DIAGNOSIS

- **Developmental delay,** as children with developmental delay may engage in self-injurious behavior or self-stimulatory behaviors, usually also seen during the day.
- **Medical disorders,** including neurologic disorders, blindness, ear infections, pain, and gastroesophageal reflux, may result in headbanging or bodyrocking.
- **Seizures,** although usually these can be easily differentiated by clinical history.

MANAGEMENT

When to Refer

If symptoms of other underlying sleep disrupters (e.g., obstructive sleep apnea) are present, the patient should be referred to a sleep specialist. Where there are concerns regarding similar behaviors during the daytime, a referral for a developmental assessment is warranted. Referral to a pediatric neurologist is seldom warranted except in the case of persistent or severe behaviors or if there is a concern regarding possible seizure disorder.

Treatment

Typically, little needs to be done if a child engages in rhythmic movements at sleep times, although parents should be instructed about safety, behavioral management, and, occasionally, alternative treatments. Usually, the most important aspect in management of headbanging or bodyrocking is **reassurance** to the family that this behavior is normal, common, benign, and self-limited; most children outgrow it by age 2 or 3 years.

Safety. All parents should be instructed to regularly tighten all screws and bolts on their child's crib or bed and to install guardrails on beds.

Behavioral management
- **Discontinue attempts to protect the child.** Even if the child is banging his head hard, it is unlikely that injury will occur. Installing extra bumpers on the crib or placing pillows in strategic places is usually not needed and is rarely effective.
- **Avoid reinforcement of the behavior.** If the parents respond to the child, they may be inadvertently reinforcing the behavior. In these cases, it may be best for the parents to ignore the behavior both at bedtime and throughout the night.
- **Dampen the noise.** Moving the crib or bed away from the wall and oiling screws and bolts can dampen noise.
- **Increase sleep.** Increasing naptimes and moving bedtime earlier may result in diminished sleep deprivation, minimizing the rhythmic behaviors related to increased nighttime arousals.

Additional treatment
- **Treat underlying sleep disrupters** (e.g., sleep disordered breathing). This may significantly decrease the frequency and duration of the rhythmic behavior.
- **Treat concurrent medical problems** (e.g., ear infections).
- **Consider pharmacologic treatment.** In severe or extremely persistent cases, treatment with a benzodiazepine may be appropriate, especially in combination with extinction if there is an attentional component. Hydroxyzine and tricyclic antidepressants have also been used for severe cases. At times, a short course of 2 to 3 weeks may be enough to disrupt the habit basis of these behaviors.

PROGNOSIS

Most young children outgrow rhythmic behaviors by age 3 years (disappear in 90% of children by age 4 years), although some children continue to engage in these behaviors throughout childhood, adolescence, and even into adulthood.

Tips for Talking to Parents

- **Explain the nature of rhythmic behaviors,** emphasizing that these are soothing behaviors for the child, similar to thumbsucking.
- **Review any factors that may be increasing difficulties falling asleep and/or nighttime arousals,** including parental attention and any sleep disrupters (e.g., sleep disordered breathing, reflux, pain).
- **Encourage parents to ignore the behavior** so that the behavior is not reinforced and maintained by parental attention.
- **Review safety issues,** including tightening of crib/bed bolts.
- **Discuss measures to reduce impact on other family members' sleep,** such as moving the crib or bed away from the wall and using white noise to mask sound.
- **Discuss the risks and benefits of treatment options,** if medication is being considered.

See Appendix F7 for parent handout on headbanging and bodyrocking.

12

Bruxism

Bruxism is the repetitive grinding or clenching of the teeth during sleep, involving both rhythmic chewing movements and periods of isotonic jaw muscle contractions. The sound of the teeth grinding, although not always audible, can be disturbing to others and is often the reason for parental concern. Bruxism can eventually lead to dental erosion, jaw pain, or tissue damage over time, although these are unlikely to be the presenting complaints in children and adolescents.

Bruxism

Bruxism is the repetitive grinding or clenching of teeth during sleep.

EPIDEMIOLOGY

Studies indicate that 70% to 90% of individuals grind their teeth to some degree during their lifetime, although it is problematic in only 5% of the population. Adult-type bruxism usually begins in late childhood or adolescence. The prevalence of bruxism increases in middle childhood, then often resolves with the eruption of the secondary dentition. One study based on parental report indicated that between 14% to 20% of children under the age of 11 years grind their teeth. In addition, approximately 50% of normal infants have bruxism following eruption of the deciduous incisors. This type of bruxism during infancy, with a median age of onset at 10.5 months, is not considered to be clinically significant. Bruxism appears to occur with equal frequency in boys and girls.

ETIOLOGY/RISK FACTORS

- **Anxiety and stress** have been linked to bruxism, which may be seen in older children and adolescents.
- **Occlusal discrepancies,** such as malocclusion and dental trauma, may increase the risk of bruxism.

- **Allergies** have been reported to be associated with bruxism.
- **Cerebral palsy and mental retardation** result in increased risk for bruxism.
- **Alcohol and stimulant medications,** such as amphetamines, can also exacerbate bruxism. Bruxism has also been reported in association with treatment with serotonin reuptake inhibitors.
- **Primary sleep disturbances** may trigger bruxism. The most destructive teeth grinding seems to occur in REM sleep.

PRESENTATION

Bruxism is characterized by clenching, gnashing, or grinding of the teeth during the night, which may be observed and/or heard by parents or others who share a bedroom with the child or adolescent. Most children with bruxism are not aware of the behavior.

Associated Features

- **Muscle pain.** Children may complain of painful and swollen jaw (masseter and temporal) muscles, limited jaw opening, or a "clicking" jaw. Bruxism can also lead to temporomandibular joint disorders.
- **Headache.** Children or adolescents with bruxism may complain of neck and shoulder pain, or headache in the morning.
- **Sensitive teeth.** Patients may complain of tooth discomfort associated with extremes in food temperature.
- **Daytime bruxism.** Children and adolescents may also grind their teeth during the day, although these two behaviors appear to be etiologically different.
- **Dental damage.** Dental damage can include erosion of the teeth, damage to the tissues surrounding the teeth (recession and inflammation of the gums), and resorption of the alveolar bone.

Diagnostic Criteria

See Table 12.1.

TABLE 12.1. *Sleep bruxism (306.8)*

Diagnostic criteria:
A. The patient has a complaint of teeth grinding or teeth clenching during sleep.
B. One or more of the following occur:
  1. Abnormal wear of the teeth
  2. Sounds associated with the bruxism
  3. Jaw muscle discomfort
C. Polysomnographic monitoring demonstrates both of the following:
  1. Jaw muscle activity during the sleep period
  2. Absence of associated epileptic activity
D. No other medical or mental disorders (e.g., sleep-related epilepsy) accounts for the abnormal movements during sleep.
E. Other sleep disorders (e.g., obstructive sleep apnea syndrome) can be present concurrently.

Minimal criteria: A plus B.
Used with permission from American Academy of Sleep Medicine. *The international classification of sleep disorders, revised: diagnostic and coding manual.* Westchester, IL: AASM, 1997:184.

EVALUATION

- **Medical history:** Generally unremarkable, but may include symptoms of head and jaw pain, dental problems.
- **Developmental/school history:** Usually normal.
- **Family history:** May be positive for other family members with bruxism.
- **Behavioral assessment:** Possible contributory factors, such as anxiety and stress, should be carefully assessed.
- **Physical examination:** Evaluation for dental erosion and tissue damage should be conducted.
- **Diagnostic tests:** Not indicated.

DIFFERENTIAL DIAGNOSIS

Diagnosis of bruxism is usually straightforward. Differential diagnosis includes:

- **Dental disorders and temporomandibular joint disorders.**
- **Seizure disorder.** In rare cases, the jaw movements may be associated with partial complex or generalized seizures.

MANAGEMENT

When to Refer

Children or adolescents with bruxism who also have significant psychiatric or behavioral issues should be referred to a mental health professional. In addition, referral to a dentist is appropriate if there are any dental concerns.

Treatment

Because bruxism is usually self-limited, treatment in children and adolescents is rarely warranted. However, since stress is a major contributing factor in many cases, possible sources of stress should be explored and eliminated if possible. Specific stress management techniques that have been shown to be helpful include the introduction of relaxing bedtime rituals, progressive relaxation exercises, hypnotherapy, and biofeedback. In more problematic cases, additional management strategies may include:

- **Sleeping position.** Lying in the supine position with support for the neck may alleviate muscle strain on the jaw and neck.
- **Pain relief.** Nonsteroidal antiinflammatory medications are occasionally indicated to relieve jaw pain. Local application of heat may be helpful.
- **Dental appliances.** For children and adolescents with dental damage or persistent complaints of jaw pain, referral to a dentist for a nighttime intraoral appliance may be warranted.

- **Pharmacotherapy.** Although REM-suppressing antidepressants have been shown to be effective for severe bruxism in adults, their use is rarely indicated in the pediatric population.
- **Psychological treatment.** If an underlying anxiety disorder is suspected, psychological treatment may be warranted.

PROGNOSIS

Bruxism, although most often self-limited in children, may be chronic and is likely to be exacerbated by stress.

Tips for Talking to Parents

- **Explain what bruxism is** in simple terms, including the long-term possibility of dental damage in older children and adolescents.
- **Explain risk factors** for bruxism, primarily stress.
- **Discuss treatment options,** if warranted, including stress management and/or psychological treatment.
- **Refer for a dental examination** in older children and adolescents.

See Appendix F8 for parent handout on bruxism.

13

Obstructive Sleep Apnea and Sleep Disordered Breathing

Obstructive sleep apnea (OSA) is a respiratory sleep disorder that is characterized by repeated episodes of prolonged upper airway obstruction during sleep. Episodes of upper airway obstruction result in complete (apnea) or partial (hypopnea) cessation of airflow at the nose and/or mouth. Multiple arousals resulting from these obstructive events lead to sleep fragmentation and frequent sleep stage transitions, and, consequently, to symptoms of daytime sleepiness (Fig. 13.1).

Obstructive Sleep Apnea

Obstructive sleep apnea is a common sleep disorder in children and adolescents that is characterized by repeated episodes of prolonged partial or complete upper airway obstruction during sleep. The obstruction is most often related to adenotonsillar hypertrophy. Multiple arousals resulting from these obstructive events lead to sleep fragmentation and, consequently, to symptoms of daytime sleepiness that often are neurobehavioral.

DEFINITION OF TERMS

- **Apnea:** discrete pauses in breathing, with duration greater than 10 seconds (or two respiratory cycle lengths in children)
- **Hypopnea:** 30% to 50% reduction in airflow
- **Obstructive apnea**: cessation of airflow accompanied by respiratory effort.
- **Central apnea**: cessation of airflow with no respiratory effort

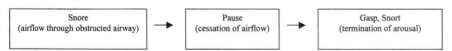

FIG. 13.1. Obstructive events resulting in multiple arousals.

- **Mixed apnea**: apnea with central and obstructive components
- **Arousal**: 3 seconds of wake electroencephalography
- **Awakenings**: 5 minutes of wake electroencephalography

CLINICAL PATTERNS OF SLEEP-DISORDERED BREATHING

It is important to understand that obstructive sleep apnea is at one end of a clinical spectrum of sleep disordered breathing that includes the following clinical conditions:

- **Primary snoring:** defined as an attempt to breathe in the face of increased upper airway resistance *without* apnea, hypopnea, or hypoxemia, or significant arousals.
- **Upper airway resistance syndrome:** characterized by increasing negative intrathoracic pressure during inspiration, as measured by balloon esophageal manometry. Arousals terminate the negative pressure swings, which results in sleep fragmentation and daytime symptoms of sleepiness. Symptoms of upper airway resistance syndrome include snoring and increased respiratory effort (including paradoxical inward rib cage movements) *without* a significant decrease in airflow or ventilatory abnormalities.
- **Partial obstructive hypoventilationhypopneas:** characterized by snoring, increased respiratory effort, and arousals, resulting in sleep disturbance and daytime symptoms *with* ventilatory abnormalities, including phasic O_2 desaturation and hypercapnea.
- **Obstructive sleep apnea:** characterized by snoring, apneic pauses, and arousals, resulting in sleep disturbance and daytime symptoms *with* ventilatory abnormalities resulting from the complete cessation of airflow.

American Academy of Pediatrics Clinical Practice Guidelines for Obstructive Sleep Apnea Syndrome (April 2002)

1. All children should be screened for snoring.
2. Complex high-risk patients should be referred to a specialist.
3. Patients with cardiorespiratory failure cannot await elective evaluation.
4. Diagnostic evaluation is useful in discriminating between primary snoring and obstructive sleep apnea syndrome, the gold standard being polysomnography.
5. Adenotonsillectomy is the first line of treatment for most children, and continuous positive airway pressure (CPAP) is an option for those who are not candidates for surgery or do not respond to surgery.
6. High-risk patients should be monitored as inpatients postoperatively.
7. Patients should be reevaluated postoperatively to determine whether additional treatment is required.

EPIDEMIOLOGY

Obstructive sleep apnea. Obstructive sleep apnea occurs in 1% to 3% of children of preschool age (little prevalence data are available for other age groups) with the following demographics:

- **Age.** Obstructive sleep apnea occurs in all ages but peaks between 2 and 6 years, coinciding with the peak age of lymphoid hyperplasia and adenotonsillar hypertrophy. A second peak occurs during adolescence, which more closely resembles "adult" obstructive sleep apnea in terms of risk factors (e.g., obesity) and clinical presentation (e.g., snoring, apnea, hypersomnolence).
- **Gender.** Obstructive sleep apnea has an equal distribution in prepubertal children, with an increased prevalence in boys after puberty that is similar to adult distribution. However, some studies have suggested a male preponderance even in younger children.
- **Ethnicity.** Some data suggest that African American children may have a higher risk.
- **Family history.** Positive family history of obstructive sleep apnea or disruptive snoring is found in a significant percentage of children with obstructive sleep apnea symptoms.

Primary snoring. Primary snoring occurs *occasionally* in 20% of children and *habitually* (nightly) in 10% (range: 3% to 12%).

ETIOLOGY/RISK FACTORS

There are a number of factors that put a child at risk for obstructive sleep apnea, although the primary risk factor in most children is adenotonsillar hypertrophy. In general terms, obstructive sleep apnea is usually related to some combination of *decreased upper airway patency* (upper airway obstruction), *reduced capacity to maintain airway patency* (decreased upper airway diameter and muscle tone), and *decreased drive to breathe* in the face of reduced upper airway patency (reduced central ventilatory drive).

Underlying mechanisms. Specific factors related to these underlying mechanisms include:

- **Upper airway obstruction** varies in degree and level (i.e., nose, nasal/oropharynx, craniofacial). Underlying obstruction may be due to:
  - Adenotonsillar hypertrophy, although tonsillar size does not necessarily correlate with degree of obstruction.
  - Allergies associated with chronic rhinitis/nasal obstruction.
  - Asthma.
  - Gastroesophageal reflux (due to pharyngeal edema).
  - Velopharyngeal flap cleft palate repair.
- **Upper airway size and muscle tone** (i.e., a small or "floppy" airway) also has an important role in the underlying pathophysiology of obstructive sleep apnea. Factors that may influence patency of the upper airway include:
  - Obesity.

- Prader-Willi syndrome (hypotonia).
- Neuromuscular disease, including hypotonic cerebral palsy and muscular dystrophies.
- Hypothyroidism (mechanism may also be related to reduced upper airway patency or reduced central ventilatory drive).
- **Central ventilatory drive** may be reduced in some children with obstructive sleep apnea. Conditions that may be associated with reduction in drive include:
  - Arnold-Chiari syndrome type II.
  - Myelomeningocele.
  - Brainstem injury or masses.
- **Combination of risk factors** is common. Down syndrome is a classic example in which multiple risk factors for obstructive sleep apnea are commonly present, such as hypotonia, glossoptosis (posterior tongue displacement), obesity, midface hypoplasia, and increased risk of lower respiratory tract anomalies and hypothyroidism.

Medical conditions. Obviously, there are a host of medical conditions occurring in children that share some of these specific risk factors. Table 13.1 lists the most common medical conditions in children that are associated with increased risk for obstructive sleep apnea.

Obesity. Although most children with obstructive sleep apnea are of normal weight, a substantial percentage are overweight or obese, and many of these children are school aged and younger. Given the epidemic of childhood obesity in our society, that number is likely to increase. An increase in the amount of adipose tissue in the throat (pharyngeal fat pads), neck (increased neck circumference), and chest wall creates increased upper airway resistance and increased work of breathing. There may be a component of altered central ventilatory drive as well. These children and adolescents are at substantial risk for perioperative complications during surgery and for associated obstructive sleep apnea conditions such as systemic hypertension.

TABLE 13.1. *Medical conditions associated with obstructive sleep apnea in children*

Craniofacial syndromes:	Miscellaneous disorders:
Midfacial hypoplasia:	Obesity
Apert syndrome	Prader-Willi syndrome
Crouzon syndrome	Hypothyroid
Pfeiffer syndrome	Mucopolysaccaridoses
Treacher-Collins	Sickle cell disease
Macroglossia/glossoptosis:	Choanal stenosis
Down syndrome	Laryngomalacia
Beckwith-Wiedemann syndrome	Airway papillomatosis
Pierre Robin syndrome	Subglottic stenosis
Neurological disorders:	Other syndromes:
Cerebral palsy	Achondroplasia
Myasthenia gravis	Hallerman-Streiff syndrome
Mobius syndrome	Klippel-Feil syndrome
Arnold-Chiari malformation	Goldenhar syndrome
Meningomyelocele	Marfan syndrome

TABLE 13.2. *Comparison between children and adults with obstructive sleep apnea*

Factor	Children	Adults
Demographics:		
Estimated prevalence	1%–2%	2%–4%
Peak age	2–6 yr	30–60 yr
Gender	M/F 1:1	M/F 8–10:1
Weight	Normal, FTT, overweight	Overweight
Major cause	Enlarged T & A	Obesity
Associated disorders	Craniofacial anomaly, neurologic disorders	Post-menopausal
Polysomnography:		
Gas-exchange abnormalities	Frequent	Usually
Duration of obstructive apneas	Any	>10 sec
Abnormal apnea index	>1	>5
Abnormal RDI	>5	>10
Sleep architecture	Often normal	Abnormal
Movement/arousal	Occasional	Common

FTT, failure to thrive; RDI, respiratory disturbance index; T & A, tonsils and adenoids.

The Obesity Epidemic and Obstructive Sleep Apnea

As the prevalence of childhood obesity increases, weight is likely to become more of a relative risk factor for pediatric obstructive sleep apnea. Practitioners should periodically screen for obstructive sleep apnea symptoms in children who are overweight or obese.

PRESENTATION/SYMPTOMS

Presentation

The most common presenting complaints in childhood obstructive sleep apnea are loud snoring, breathing pauses, and difficulty breathing during sleep. Obstructive sleep apnea is unlikely in the absence of habitual snoring, although many children who snore do not have obstructive sleep apnea. However, parents may not spontaneously volunteer information about obstructive sleep apnea symptoms, such as snoring, and the history may only be elicited on direct questioning (a screening questionnaire for obstructive sleep apnea is provided in Appendix C). In addition, because obstructive sleep apnea may occur primarily during REM sleep, which is concentrated in the last third of the night, parents may not be awake to observe the most severe symptoms. Finally, parents of adolescents may be less likely to observe and note snoring and disturbed sleep.

Because parents do not necessarily associate behavior and academic problems with sleep problems, concerns such as hyperactivity, impulsivity, and irritability may be the presenting complaints for obstructive sleep apnea in children.

Symptoms

Common presenting symptoms of pediatric obstructive sleep apnea include:

Nocturnal symptoms:
- **Loud, continuous nightly snoring,** although volume does not necessarily correlate with the degree of obstruction.
- **Apneic pauses,** although more commonly parents may describe episodic choking, gasping, and snorting during the night. There is often increased parental anxiety about sleep respirations.
- **Paradoxical movement** of chest wall and abdomen during breathing.
- **Restless sleep,** thrashing, and increased body movement.
- **Sweating** during sleep, related to increased work of breathing.
- **Abnormal sleeping position,** such as propped on pillows or sleeping with the neck hyperextended.

Daytime symptoms:
- **Mouth breathing,** due to adenoidal hypertrophy, and dry mouth.
- **Chronic nasal congestion/rhinorrhea.**
- **Hyponasal speech.**
- **Difficulty swallowing,** related to tonsillar hypertrophy.
- **Morning headaches** that may be related to CO_2 retention.
- **Frequent infections,** especially otitis media and sinusitis.
- **Poor appetite,** which may be related to dysphagia and chronic nasal obstruction.

Excessive daytime sleepiness, which may present with more "classic" symptoms of hypersomnolence:
- **Difficulty waking** in the morning.
- **Falling asleep** in school or at inappropriate times.
- **Increased nap** need in younger children.

And/or may present with more subtle neurobehavioral signs (especially in younger children):
- **Mood changes,** such as irritability, low frustration tolerance, impatience, mood swings, depression/anxiety, and social withdrawal.
- **Acting-out behaviors,** including aggression and hyperactivity.
- **Inattention,** poor concentration, and distractibility.
- **"ADHD"**-like symptoms.
- **Academic problems.**

Playing Detective

Obstructive sleep apnea in children may present solely with parental complaints of behavior problems, inattentiveness ("ADHD"), and academic failure. Parents may not volunteer information about sleep and symptoms of sleep disordered breathing (snoring) unless these are directly elicited by the primary care provider.

TABLE 13.3. *Diagnostic criteria: obstructive sleep apnea syndrome (780.53-0)*

A. The patient has a complaint of excessive sleepiness or insomnia. Occasionally, the patient may be unaware of clinical features that are observed by others.
B. Frequent episodes of obstructed breathing during sleep.
C. Associated features include:
    1. Loud snoring
    2. Morning headaches
    3. A dry mouth upon waking
    4. Chest retraction during sleep in young children
D. Polysomnographic monitoring demonstrates:
    1. More than five obstructive apneas, greater than 10 seconds in duration, per hour of sleep and one or more of the following:
        a. Frequent arousals from sleep associated with the apneas
        b. Bradytachycardia
        c. Arterial oxygen desaturation in association with the apneic episodes
    2. An MSLT that demonstrates a mean sleep latency of less than 10 minutes.
E. Can be associated with other medical disorders, e.g., tonsillar enlargement.
F. Other sleep disorders can be present, e.g., periodic limb movement disorder or narcolepsy.

Minimal criteria: A plus B plus C.
MSLT, multiple sleep latency test.
Used with permission from American Academy of Sleep Medicine. *The international classification of sleep disorders, revised: diagnostic and coding manual.* Westchester, IL: AASM, 1997: 57–58.

Associated Features

- **Enuresis** (especially secondary), due to alterations in antidiuretic hormone secretion related to disturbed sleep.
- **Growth failure** (in severe cases, failure to thrive) that may be related to some combination of decreased appetite and decreased intake, increased metabolic needs from increased work of breathing, and alterations in normal nocturnal growth hormone secretion patterns.
- **Increase in partial arousal parasomnias** (e.g., sleepwalking, sleep terrors) in susceptible children, which is related to sleep fragmentation and increased slow-wave sleep.
- **Increase in seizure frequency** in predisposed children, which is possibly related to increased arousals and intermittent hypoxia.
- **Behavioral sleep problems,** such as bedtime resistance and nightwakings, occurring in as many as 25% of children with primary obstructive sleep apnea. These sleep problems may be secondary to the obstructive sleep apnea (sleep fragmentation related to arousals resulting in more nightwakings) or exist independently.

EVALUATION

Evaluation for obstructive sleep apnea includes history of signs and symptoms, physical examination, and overnight polysomnography. It is important to note that no combination of symptoms and physical findings has been found that reliably distinguishes obstructive sleep apnea from primary snoring.

- **Medical history:** Both medical risk factors for and medical sequelae of obstructive sleep apnea may be present. The history is often positive for both upper airway (chronic sinusitis) and lower airway (asthma) disease, allergies, and frequent upper respiratory infections. There may be a history of frequent episodes of streptococcal pharyngitis/tonsillitis. Symptoms suggestive of gastroesophageal reflux (heartburn, vomiting) should be elicited.
- **Developmental/school history:** Although the developmental/school history may be normal, there is frequently a history of significant academic concerns, as well as attentional and learning problems. Certain syndromes with developmental delay as a prominent feature (e.g., Down syndrome, Prader-Willi syndrome) are associated with increased risk for obstructive sleep apnea.
- **Family history:** Often positive for diagnosed obstructive sleep apnea, as well as loud snoring.
- **Behavioral assessment:** Evaluation of behavioral and mood concerns is key in assessing the extent of daytime sleepiness–related sequelae.
- **Physical examination:** In the majority of cases, the physical examination of children with obstructive sleep apnea is completely normal. However, the primary care clinician should assess for the following:
  - **Growth:** including overweight and obesity, as well as failure to thrive (especially in younger children).
  - **Head, eyes, ears, nose, throat (HEENT):**
    - **Facial structure:** "adenoidal facies" midface hypoplasia, retro- and micrognathia.
    - **Signs of atopy:** including "allergic shiners," nasal crease ("allergic salute"), and eczema.
    - **Mouth breathing:** may indicate enlarged adenoids and/or chronic congestion.
    - **Hyponasality:** ask child to repeat "Mickey Mouse," "ninety-nine," or "my name is money" while occluding the nose; a child with significant nasal obstruction will sound the same with occlusion as without.
    - **Nasal passage patency** and **septal deviation:** including edematous turbinates and nasal polyps.
    - **Oropharyngeal examination:** including tongue size, palatal integrity, tonsillar size, size of the uvula, and posterior pharyngeal space (Fig. 13.2).

Size Doesn't Count, After All

A number of studies have shown that there is no reliable relationship between the size of the tonsils and adenoids and the presence of obstructive sleep apnea confirmed by polysomnography. Children with impressive adenotonsillar hypertrophy may not have obstructive sleep apnea, and children with small tonsils and adenoids may have significant obstruction.

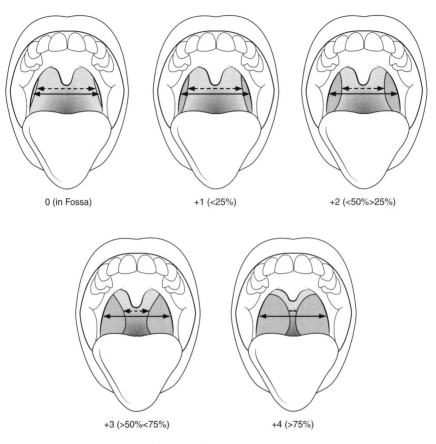

FIG. 13.2. Grading tonsillar size.

- **Neck examination:** assess for thyromegaly, as hypothyroidism appears to be a risk factor for obstructive sleep apnea, at least in adults.
- **Cardiac examination:** for signs of pulmonary hypertension and resulting cor pulmonale (such as loud S_2, systolic murmur, and displaced point of maximum impulse). Fortunately, these signs of severe obstructive sleep apnea are now rarely seen. There may be systemic hypertension, although this is much less common in children than in adults.

Why a Sleep Study?

Although history and physical examination are important in making the diagnosis of obstructive sleep apnea in children, *no combination of symptoms and physical findings has been found that reliably distinguishes obstructive sleep apnea from primary snoring.* Overnight polysomnography remains the diagnostic gold standard.

Diagnostic Tests

For the most part, laboratory studies are unnecessary in obstructive sleep apnea, although in severe cases polycythemia and/or metabolic alkalosis may be noted.

Radiologic Studies/Electrocardiography

- An upright lateral neck x-ray to evaluate for hypertrophy of the tonsils/adenoids and upper airway patency may be warranted. Cephalometric radiographs may be helpful in assessing the upper airway structure in children with craniofacial anomalies but are seldom necessary in normal children.
- In cases of severe obstructive sleep apnea, there may be evidence of right ventricular hypertrophy on chest x-ray. The electrocardiogram may also show evidence of right ventricular enlargement.

Polysomnography: The Gold Standard

At the present time, given that the only way to make a definitive diagnosis of obstructive sleep apnea is with overnight polysomnography, a sleep study should be performed in every child with significant nocturnal and diurnal symptoms and risk factors for obstructive sleep apnea (see Chapter 4 for more information on overnight polysomnography). Figure 13.3 depicts an apneic event with a consequent decrease in oxygen saturation.

American Thoracic Society's Indications for Cardiopulmonary Sleep Studies in Children

- **Differentiate benign snoring** from snoring associated with sleep disordered breathing.
- **Assess severity** of obstructive sleep apnea.
- **Clarify diagnosis** when symptoms and risk factors are discordant.
- **Screen children at high risk** for obstructive sleep apnea (e.g., trisomy 21, achondroplasia).
- **Delineate severity of obstructive sleep apnea** in children at risk for peri- and postoperative symptoms.
- **Titrate CPAP** in children with diagnosed obstructive sleep apnea.

Polysomnography is also important as a baseline measure for children with additional risk factors in whom obstructive sleep apnea is not likely to completely resolve with adenotonsillectomy alone (e.g., obesity, craniofacial anomalies), and who therefore may need a follow-up postoperative sleep study.

Other "screening" studies thus far appear to have limited usefulness in children (home audio/videotaping, overnight oximetry) as do shortened polysomographic or "nap" studies because they are likely to underestimate the presence

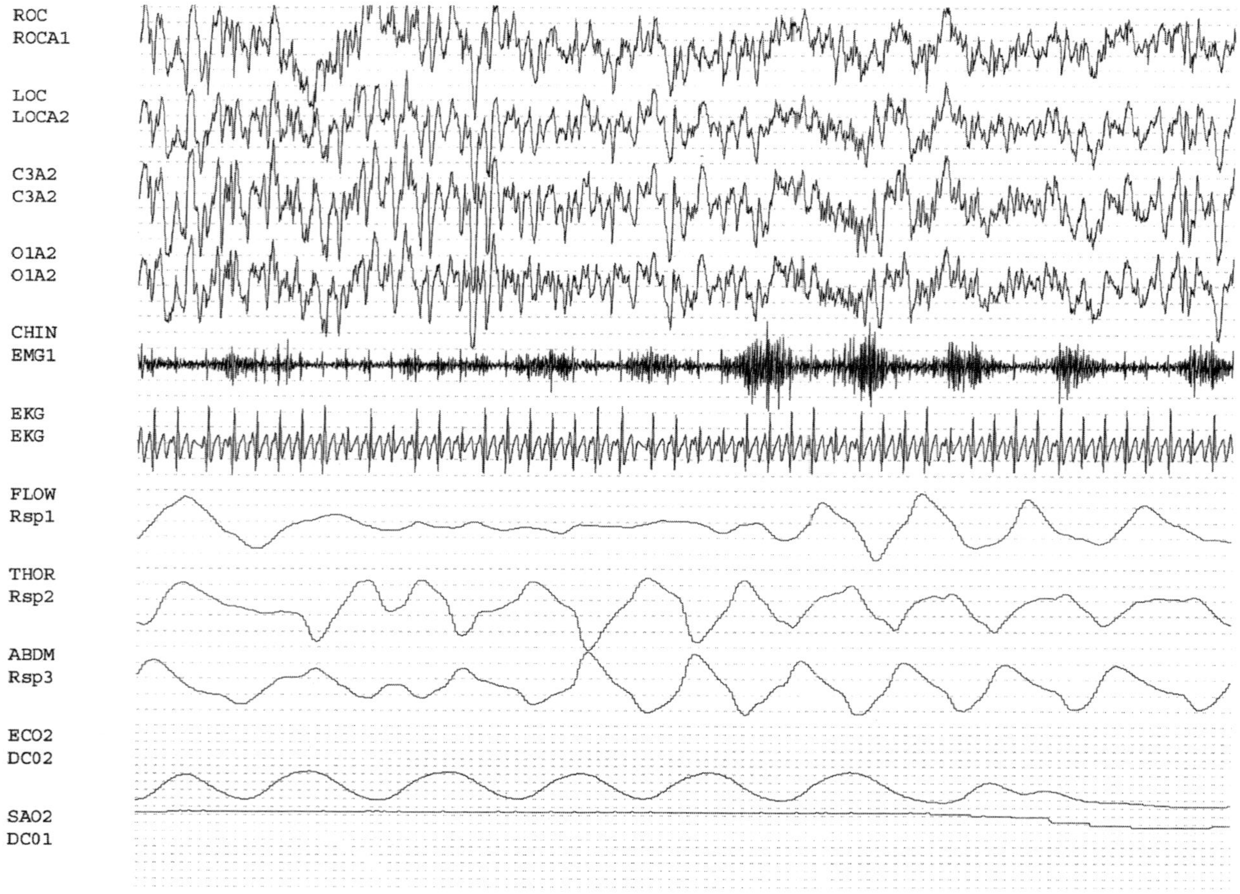

ROC
ROCA1

LOC
LOCCA2

C3A2
C3A2

O1A2
O1A2

CHIN
EMG1

EKG
EKG

FLOW
Rsp1

THOR
Rsp2

ABDM
Rsp3

ECO2
DCO2

SAO2
DC01

FIG. 13.3. Obstructive sleep apnea.

and severity of disease. These types of studies are helpful if the results are positive (high positive predictive value) but warrant corroboration with a standard overnight sleep study if the results are negative (low negative predictive value).

Transesophageal balloon manometry is performed in some sleep labs to detect upper airway resistance syndrome, especially in the face of significant obstructive sleep apnea symptoms with a normal sleep study. However, esophageal pressure monitoring is expensive and often not well tolerated by children; thus, it is not currently considered a standard part of the overnight sleep study evaluation.

The polysomnography parameter most commonly used in evaluating for sleep-disordered breathing is the *apnea/hypopnea index (AHI)*, which indicates the number of apneic and hypopneic events per hour of sleep. The AHI may include central events (which may normally occur during sleep at all ages, especially in REM sleep, and at the transition from wake to sleep or from one sleep stage to another), as well as mixed and obstructive events. The *apnea index (AI)* is the number of apneic-only events per hour. The *sleep stage distribution* of events (often significantly increased during REM sleep) and *relationship to sleeping position* (frequently increased in the supine position) should also be noted. The *arousal index* (number of arousals per hour of sleep), particularly the arousals related to respiratory events index, is also important as an indicator of the degree of sleep fragmentation resulting from obstructive respiratory events.

It should be noted that currently there are no *universally* accepted polysomnographic parameters for diagnosing obstructive sleep apnea in children, and it is still unclear which parameters predict morbidity. Therefore, the following definitions are based on commonly accepted consensus criteria:

- **AHI ≥ 5 or AI > 1.** Unlike adults, obstructive apneas in normal children are rare; therefore, most pediatric pulmonologists consider an apnea index (AI) >1 to be abnormal. In cases in which the AHI is between 1 and 5 obstructive events per hour (the "gray zone"), clinical judgment regarding risk factors for obstructive sleep apnea, evidence of daytime sequelae, and the technical quality of the overnight sleep study should determine further management. In some cases, it may be prudent to consider repeating the sleep study if the clinical index of suspicion remains high in the face of a negative study.
- **O_2 desaturation nadir <92%.**
- **Change in nadir O_2 from baseline > 4%.**
- **Maximal end-tidal CO_2 > 53.**
- **Increased end-tidal CO_2 > 45 for >60% of total sleep time (TST).**

DIFFERENTIAL DIAGNOSIS

- **Excessive daytime sleepiness** can result from other sleep disorders, including narcolepsy, idiopathic hypersomnolence, insufficient sleep syndrome, and periodic limb movement disorder. Daytime sleepiness can also be related to psychiatric disorders, such as depression, and medical conditions.

- **Respiratory disturbance** can be due to central sleep apnea, primary snoring, paroxysmal nocturnal dyspnea, or asthma.
- **Movements,** as well as respiratory disturbances associated with nocturnal seizures, may mimic obstructive sleep apnea–related gasping and arousals.
- **Upper airway obstruction** may be related to laryngomalacia, vascular ring, or gastroesophageal reflux.

MANAGEMENT

When to Refer

When there are straightforward obstructive sleep apnea symptoms (e.g., snoring, apneic pauses) with clear-cut risk factors (e.g., adenotonsillar hypertrophy) in an otherwise healthy child, the primary care pediatrician may be comfortable referring for and interpreting the result of the overnight sleep study. However, in cases in which there are additional risk factors (e.g., obesity, congenital syndromes), evidence of severe disease (e.g., growth failure, significant neurobehavioral sequelae), or other complicating factors (e.g., underlying medical conditions), consultation with a sleep center that has pediatric expertise is warranted. In addition, children who are candidates for CPAP treatment should be referred to a pediatric sleep center.

Treatment

The decision of whether to treat obstructive sleep apnea and how is contingent on the severity (symptoms, sleep study results, and complications), duration, and underlying etiologic factors in a given child.

- **AHI > 10:** In the case of moderate to severe disease, the decision to treat is usually straightforward.
- **AHI between 5 and 10:** Because the long-term neurobehavioral and cognitive consequences of even mild obstructive sleep apnea are not known, most pediatric sleep experts believe that any child with an apnea index > 5 and/or O_2 desaturation $< 85\%$ should be treated.
- **AHI between 1 and 5:** For an apnea index between 1 and 5, the decision to treat is based on the presence or absence of other clinical sequelae (e.g., excessive daytime sleepiness, neurobehavioral complications).

Treatment options include:

- **Adenotonsillectomy** is the most common treatment for pediatric obstructive sleep apnea and the first-line treatment in any child with significant adenotonsillar hypertrophy, even in the presence of additional risk factors such as obesity. Adenotonsillectomy in uncomplicated cases generally (70% to 90% of children) results in complete resolution of symptoms. Removal of both the tonsils and adenoids is recommended to avoid recurrence of symptoms, even if one appears to be the primary abnormality (regrowth of adenoidal tissue, even after surgical removal, also occurs in some cases).

Peri- and postoperative complications, especially respiratory compromise, are more common in general in children with obstructive sleep apnea (as high as 25%). Other potential complications include hemorrhage, pain, and poor oral intake with dehydration. Groups considered high-risk include:

- Children **younger than 3 years.**
- Children with **severe obstructive sleep apnea,** as documented by polysomnography.
- Children who already have **significant clinical sequelae** of obstructive sleep apnea (e.g., failure to thrive).
- Children with **associated medical conditions,** such as craniofacial syndromes, morbid obesity, and hypotonia.

Relative contraindications to adenotonsillectomy include children with cleft palate and velopharyngeal insufficiency, as well as submucous cleft.

Both the surgeon and the anesthesiologist should be provided with information on the child's apnea, as well as with the results of the sleep study. Careful postoperative monitoring is recommended for children with obstructive sleep apnea. Some centers have adopted a policy that all children undergoing adenotonsillectomy for obstructive sleep apnea should be monitored overnight, as the immediate postoperative period may not have adequate REM sleep in which to observe worsening of any ventilatory abnormalities. Children with severe disease should be monitored in an intensive care setting.

Due to postoperative edema, obstructive sleep apnea symptoms may take 6 to 8 weeks to completely resolve. All patients should be reevaluated postoperatively to determine whether additional treatment is required. If there are significant residual risk factors or continued symptoms, a follow-up sleep study at least 6 weeks post adenotonsillectomy may be indicated.

- **Other surgical procedures,** such as nasal septoplasty, epiglottoplasty, uvulopharyngopalatoplasty, and maxillofacial surgery, are seldom performed in children but may be indicated in selected cases. Tracheotomy is rarely indicated, except in the case of severe, life-threatening obstructive sleep apnea.
- **CPAP (or bilevel positive airway pressure, BiPAP)** is the most common treatment for obstructive sleep apnea in adults. CPAP is a noninvasive method of providing distending pressure to maintain a patent upper airway. CPAP can be used successfully with children and adolescents, even children as young as a year old. It should be considered a palliative rather than a curative therapy, and may be needed for a prolonged period of time. CPAP may be indicated in the following clinical situations:
  - Adenotonsillectomy not indicated or contraindicated.

- Adenotonsillectomy fails to completely resolve symptoms, usually in children with additional risk factors such as obesity, craniofacial anomalies, or trisomy 21.
- Prior to surgery in children with severe obstructive sleep apnea.

CPAP involves a nasal mask or facemask that is securely attached by velcro straps and special head gear (there may be an increased risk of aspiration in children with full face masks). It is important to ensure a tight seal without air leaks; a chin strap may be added to prevent air leaks through the mouth. Optimal pressure settings (that abolish or minimize respiratory events without increasing arousals) are determined in the sleep lab during CPAP titration and should be retitrated periodically (at least yearly or with significant weight changes) with long-term use. Potential side effects from CPAP use include nasal congestion, dryness, and rhinorrhea; eye irritation; and facial dermatitis. Adding warmed and humidified air and slowly increasing pressure over time ("ramp time") may alleviate some of these side effects. Patients may complain of feelings of claustrophobia and difficulty exhaling; in situations in which these problems prevent successful usage, BiPAP (which allows expiratory, as well as inspiratory pressure to be set) may be a better tolerated alternative.

Compliance with CPAP is a key factor in determining success. Adolescents pose a particular challenge. But even children with significant developmental delays or trisomy 21 can be successful CPAP users. It may be helpful to set up a behavioral program utilizing such techniques as positive reinforcement, training parents to manage resistant behavior, modeling, desensitization, and shaping, in coordination with a behavioral therapist. For many children, the dramatic improvement in quality of life with CPAP use is an important motivating factor for continued use.

- **Weight management,** including nutritional, exercise, and behavioral components, is indicated for all children with obstructive sleep apnea who are overweight or obese. Significantly compromised obese patients may benefit from an inpatient weight loss program.
- **Medications,** including nasal decongestants or nasal steroids, may be appropriate in cases in which nasal congestion and/or mild adenoidal hypertrophy are contributing factors. Sedating agents, medications containing alcohol, or medications with respiratory depressant effects should be avoided as they may exacerbate obstructive sleep apnea (see also Chapter 19). Exposure to environmental tobacco smoke and other pollutants should also be avoided.
- **Supplemental oxygen therapy is seldom warranted** in children with obstructive sleep apnea, unless there are special circumstances. In fact, oxygen therapy may worsen hypoventilation.
- **Oral appliances,** such as mandibular advancing devices and tongue retainers, are occasionally used in adolescents in whom facial bone growth is largely complete. Referral to an orthodontist specializing in these devices would be indicated in this situation.

- **Positional therapy** can be used in some patients when obstructive events are mild and worse in the supine position. A tennis ball or other firm ball may be sewn into the pocket of a pajama top or T-shirt that is worn backward to bed, preventing the child from sleeping in the supine position.
- **Treatment of coexisting sleep disorders** is important because many children with obstructive sleep apnea also have other sleep problems, including behavioral sleep disorders, that result in significant sleep deprivation or fragmentation. Complete resolution of daytime symptoms may not occur unless these are addressed as well.

PROGNOSIS

Studies suggest that for most children symptoms of obstructive sleep apnea, including learning and behavior problems, completely resolve with appropriate treatment. However, little is known about the long-term neurobehavioral consequences in untreated or partially treated children. Chronicity and severity of the obstructive sleep apnea, as well as individual factors (e.g., age, developmental level), are likely to play important roles in determining long-term effects. Children with obstructive sleep apnea initially treated successfully with adenotonsillectomy may redevelop symptoms as older children or adolescents if additional risk factors emerge (e.g., obesity). Children with obstructive sleep apnea may also be predisposed to develop the condition as adults, although no long-term prospective studies have been done.

Tips for Talking to Parents

- **Explain what obstructive sleep apnea is** in simple terms, including the associated sleep disruption (a good analogy for frequent arousals is like being poked in the arm every few seconds while you are asleep).
- **Reassure parents that their child will not stop breathing completely some day and die!**
- **Explain risk factors** for obstructive sleep apnea, primarily enlarged tonsils and adenoids. If the child is significantly overweight, address the issue up front.
- **Review the daytime consequences** of obstructive sleep apnea. Parents may not attribute hyperactivity or moodiness, for example, to a sleep problem.
- **Explain what to expect from the overnight sleep study.**
- **Review the results of the overnight sleep study.** In interpreting the study's implications, it is important to ask parents if the child's breathing was "typical" on the night of the study. Parents frequently report that their child "slept much better" in the lab!
- **Discuss the risks and benefits of treatment options,** including adenotonsillectomy, weight loss, and other treatment choices.
- **Encourage any parent who snores loudly and has daytime symptoms to be evaluated for sleep apnea.**

See Appendix F9 for parent handout on obstructive sleep apnea.

14

Restless Legs Syndrome and Periodic Limb Movement Disorder

Restless legs syndrome (RLS) is a sensorimotor disorder characterized by uncomfortable sensations in the lower extremities, usually accompanied by an almost irresistible urge to move the legs. These subjective uncomfortable and unpleasant sensations (dysasthesias) occur primarily in the legs, although sometimes the arms and other body parts are also involved. Most episodes begin during periods of rest or inactivity, such as lying in bed to fall asleep, and both the likelihood of having symptoms and the severity of symptoms tend to increase with the duration of inactivity. These sensations are usually immediately relieved by movement, including walking, rocking, or other motion, as long as the motion continues. Some patients with RLS do not describe a significant sensory component but may experience fidgetiness and leg movements during periods of rest as the primary presenting symptom.

Ironically, in RLS the conditions that produce the symptoms are the same conditions that are needed to initiate sleep (inactivity and rest); conversely, the behaviors that relieve symptoms (activity and motion) are likely to interfere with sleep onset. In children, parents may interpret these behaviors as bedtime resistance and difficulty falling asleep.

Restless Legs Syndrome

RLS is characterized by uncomfortable sensations in the legs resulting in motor restlessness to relieve the symptoms. Symptoms are worse or exclusively present at night, with temporary relief with motor activity.

Periodic Limb Movement Disorder (PLMD) is characterized by periodic, repetitive episodes of stereotyped limb movements occurring in a series of 20- to 40-second intervals during sleep. These movements usually occur in the legs and frequently consist of rhythmic extension of the big toe and dorsiflexion at the ankle. Although often associated with a partial arousal or an awakening, patients with periodic limb movements are usually unaware of them and of the sleep disruption.

Periodic Limb Movement Disorder

PLMD is characterized by periodic episodes of repetitive and stereotyped limb movements during sleep, often associated with a partial arousal or an awakening.

RLS and PLMD often occur concomitantly, and both result in sleep disruption. Studies in adults indicate that 70% to 90% of adults with RLS have PLMD; whereas only 20% of patients with PLMD have RLS. Similar studies have not been conducted with children or adolescents.

It is important to note that these two disorders have only been recently recognized in children and adolescents. Recent investigations indicate that both of these disorders are much more common in adults than previously thought, and the same is likely true in children and adolescents. Therefore, pediatric practitioners should consider RLS and PLMD in the differential diagnosis for any sleep problem that includes significant difficulties falling asleep; nighttime awakenings with restless sleep; or unexplained symptoms of daytime somnolence, including neurobehavioral symptoms (e.g., inattentiveness, irritability).

EPIDEMIOLOGY

- RLS and PLMD are common disorders in adults, although significantly underdiagnosed. In adults, RLS is found in 5% to 15% of the population. The prevalence of PLMD is positively correlated with age (5% of adults age 30 to 50, 29% in adults 50 to 64, and 44% in those older than 65). The prevalence of RLS and of PLMD in the pediatric population is unknown, although one recent study found that 17% of more than 800 children surveyed reported "restless legs at night." Furthermore, approximately 40% of adults with RLS report the onset of symptoms before age 20.
- Several studies in referral populations have found that periodic limb movements occur in as much as one fourth of children diagnosed with attention deficit-hyperactivity disorder (ADHD). Other recent studies have found an association between symptoms of hyperactivity and the presence of periodic

limb movements. It should be emphasized that the prevalence of PLMD in the general population of children with ADHD is unknown.

ETIOLOGY/RISK FACTORS

Restless Legs Syndrome

Primary RLS is idiopathic in nature.
- **Genetic link** is postulated to follow an autosomal-dominant pattern. Idiopathic cases of RLS have a high familial incidence (92%), with the prevalence of RLS in first-degree relatives of patients with early-onset RLS (age < 45 years) six to seven times that of the general population. Fifty percent to 60% of adult RLS patients have a positive family history.

Secondary RLS can occur in relation to a number of different medical conditions. In secondary cases, the symptoms generally remit when the underlying condition has resolved. These include (some of these have only been described in adults):
- **Iron deficiency anemia,** as an association between RLS and low serum ferritin levels in particular has been described in children, as well as in adults. This may occur in the face of normal hemoglobin levels. Vitamin B_{12} and folate deficiencies have also been associated with RLS.
- **Neurologic disorders,** including polyneuropathy, lumbosacral radiculopathy, and myelopathy.
- **Medical disorders,** including diabetes mellitus, end-stage renal disease, cancer, peripheral vascular disease, rheumatoid arthritis, and hypothyroidism. RLS appears to be more common in children with Williams syndrome.
- **Pregnancy,** as RLS occurs in up to 15% of pregnant women, most commonly in the last trimester. Some women (approximately 1 in 7) who develop RLS in pregnancy continue to have symptoms postpartum.
- **Drugs and chemicals,** as substances that may exacerbate underlying RLS include caffeine, alcohol, neuroleptics, metoclopramide, sedatives or narcotics (withdrawal from), lithium, calcium channel blockers, most antiemetics, phenytoin, dopamine receptor blockers, and some antidepressants.

Periodic Limb Movement Disorder

Neurophysiologic mechanisms are unknown. It is theorized that central dopamine may be involved in the pathophysiology of PLMD given the treatment efficacy of L-dopa and dopamine agonists.

Secondary PLMD can be the result of:
- **Iron deficiency anemia**
- **Metabolic disorders,** including uremia
- **Childhood leukemia**

- **Medications,** including tricyclic antidepressants, fluoxetine, and venlafaxine. Withdrawal from other medications, including anticonvulsants, benzodiazepines, and hypnotics, can exacerbate periodic limb movements.
- **Obstructive sleep apnea** and associated arousals may precipitate periodic limb movements.

PRESENTATION

- **Restless Legs Syndrome** *(a screening questionnaire for RLS is provided in Appendix D)*
  - **Sensory complaints.** Patients generally do not describe the leg sensations as painful, although younger children may not be able to articulate their specific sensory disturbances. Other complaints by the patient (or parent) may include uncomfortable sensations "inside" or deep in the legs, or "growing pains."

The Vocabulary of Restless Legs Syndrome

Patients may use a variety of descriptive terms to describe their sensory symptoms, including "creepy/crawly, "pulling," "electric current," "gotta moves," "heebie-jeebies," "itchy bones," and "crazy legs."

  - **Increased symptoms with inactivity.** Although no specific body position is associated with RLS symptoms, the activities most likely to provoke symptoms are long periods of motor inactivity combined with decreased mental activity. In milder cases, symptoms may only be precipitated by long periods of inactivity (e.g., plane flights). It is postulated that some children may experience RLS symptoms primarily during prolonged periods of sitting in school.
  - **Relief with movement.** In addition to movement, symptoms may also be relieved by counterstimulation, such as rubbing or application of hot or cold.
- **Associated Features**
  - **Difficulty falling asleep.** Because the symptoms are usually worse in the evening or during the night, this is one of the most common presenting complaints.
  - **Problems maintaining sleep.** Restless legs symptoms may occur during night awakenings.
  - **Bedtime struggles.** If bedtime resistance is the primary presenting complaint, it is also important to evaluate for other sleep disorders (such as delayed sleep phase) that may be causing delayed sleep onset. This is because in a child with primary RLS, the longer it takes to fall asleep, the greater the likelihood that RLS symptoms will occur.

- **Daytime sleepiness.** Sleep onset difficulties that lead to reduced sleep time will often result in daytime sleepiness and associated neurobehavioral symptoms (e.g., inattentiveness, poor focusing). Sleep maintenance problems related to RLS symptoms during the night may also contribute to sleepiness.
- **Periodic limb movements.** PLMD occurs in about 80% of adult patients with RLS.
- **Periodic limb movement disorder**
  - **Restlessness during sleep.** Parents may complain that the child's bedcovers are always highly disheveled during the night and in the morning.
  - **Nighttime arousals.** Nighttime awakenings and unrefreshing sleep may be reported.
  - **Periodic limb movements.** Parents may observe limb jerks during sleep, but these have not been demonstrated to be either highly sensitive or specific in making the diagnosis.
- **Associated Features**
  - **Daytime behavior problems.** Behavior problems, including mood problems and oppositional defiant behavior, may result from the frequent nighttime arousals. Explicit symptoms of excessive daytime sleepiness (dozing off) are relatively uncommon. Because parents do not necessarily associate behavior and academic problems with sleep disturbances, concerns such as hyperactivity, impulsivity, irritability, and ADHD may be the presenting complaints.
  - **RLS symptoms.** RLS may occur in patients with PLMD (about 20%).

Diagnostic Criteria

See Tables 14.1 to 14.5.

TABLE 14.1. *Common childhood symptoms of restless legs syndrome and periodic limb movement disorder*

Bedtime symptoms	Excessive daytime sleepiness
Difficulty falling asleep	Difficulty waking in the morning
Movements of the legs and/or extremities	Morning grogginess
Walking, pacing, or running about at bedtime	Falling asleep in school or at inappropriate times
Bedtime behavior problems	Increased need for naps
Leg pain	Mood changes: irritability, low frustration tolerance, impatience, mood swings, depression/anxiety, and social withdrawal
Leg discomfort	
Nocturnal symptoms	
Leg movements	
Restless sleep	
Nighttime awakenings	Acting out behaviors: aggression, hyperactivity
Daytime symptoms	
Leg movements during rest	Oppositional defiant disorder
Inability to sit still for long periods	Inattention, poor concentration, distractibility
Leg discomfort	"ADHD" symptom complex
	Academic problems

ADHD, attention deficit-hyperactivity disorder.

TABLE 14.2. *Criteria for the diagnosis of* **definite** *restless legs syndrome in children*

1. The child meets all four essential adult criteria for RLS *and*
   a. The child relates a description in his or her own words that is consistent with leg discomfort. (The child may use terms such as "oowies," "tickle,""spiders," "boo-boos," "want to run," and "a lot of energy in my legs" to describe symptoms. Use of age-appropriate descriptors is encouraged.)
   or
   b. The child meets all four essential adult criteria for RLS *and*
2. Two of three following supportive criteria are present (see below)
   Supportive criteria for the diagnosis of *definite* restless legs syndrome in children
   a. Sleep disturbance for age
   b. A biological parent or sibling has definite RLS
   c. The child has a polysommographically documented PLMS index of 5 or more per hour of sleep.

PLMS, periodic leg movement syndrome; RLS, restless legs syndrome.
From NIH/RLS Foundation Workshop. RLS: Diagnosis and Diagnostic and Epidemiological Tools. May 2002.

TABLE 14.3. *Criteria for the diagnosis of* **probable** *restless legs syndrome in children*

1. The child meets all four essential adult criteria for RLS, except criterion 4 (the urge to move or sensations are worse in the evening or at night than during the day) *and*
2. The child has a biological parent or sibling with definite RLS
   or[a]
1. The child is observed to have behavior manifestations of lower-extremity discomfort when sitting or lying, accompanied by motor movement of the affected limbs, the discomfort has characteristics of adult criteria 2, 3, and 4 (i.e., is worse during rest and inactivity, relieved by movement, and worse during the evening and at night) *and*
2. The child has a biological parent or sibling with definite RLS

RLS, restless legs syndrome.
[a]This last *probable* category is intended for young children or cognitively impaired children, who do not have sufficient language to describe the sensory component of RLS.
From NIH/RLS Foundation Workshop. RLS: Diagnosis and Diagnostic and Epidemiological Tools. May 2002.

TABLE 14.4. *Criteria for the diagnosis of* **at risk** *for restless legs syndrome in children*

1. The child has periodic limb movement disorder (for the childhood definition, please see Table 14.5) *and*
2. The child has a biological parent or sibling with definite RLS, but the child does not meet definite or probable childhood RLS definitions (as outlined above)

RLS, restless legs syndrome.
From NIH/RLS Foundation Workshop. RLS: Diagnosis and Diagnostic and Epidemiological Tools. May 2002.

TABLE 14.5. *Criteria for the diagnosis of periodic limb movement disorder in children*

1. Polysomnography shows a periodic leg movement index of 5 or more per hour of sleep. The leg movements are 0.5–5 sec in duration, arise at intervals of 5–90 sec, occur in groups of 4 or more, and have an amplitude of one-quarter or more of toe dorsiflexion during calibration *and*
2. Clinical sleep disturbance for age must be evident as manifested by sleep onset problems, sleep maintenance problems, or excessive sleepiness *and*
3. The leg movements cannot be accounted for by sleep-disordered breathing (i.e., the movements are independent of any abnormal respiratory events) or medication effect (e.g., antidepressant medication).

From NIH/RLS Foundation Workshop. RLS: Diagnosis and Diagnostic and Epidemiological Tools. May 2002.

EVALUATION

Diagnosis

The diagnosis of RLS is based solely on clinical history, whereas PLMD should be objectively quantified by an overnight sleep study (polysomnography). However, because a high percentage (80%) of RLS patients also have PLMD, the finding of periodic limb movements on overnight sleep study is also supportive of the diagnosis of RLS.

- **Medical history:** May include a history of iron deficiency anemia. Children with the medical conditions listed above are at increased risk for secondary RLS and PLMD. Concurrent medications should be reviewed as possible contributory factors. Caffeine intake may exacerbate symptoms of RLS.
- **Developmental history:** Generally benign.
- **Family history:** May not be positive for diagnosed RLS/PLMD, as these are frequently misdiagnosed in adults, but there may be a strong family history of "insomnia" or "growing pains."
- **Behavioral assessment:** May reveal significant behavior problems, mood disturbances, and ADHD.
- **Physical examination:** Generally normal (including the neurologic exam) in children with primary RLS/PLMD. However, the primary care clinician may note from behavioral observation that many children with RLS are not able to sit still for long periods and often jiggle their legs while sitting for prolonged periods.
- **Diagnostic tests:**
  - **Polysomnography:**
    - **RLS:** Although RLS is a clinical diagnosis, the presence of periodic limb movements on an overnight sleep study is helpful because of the frequent concurrence of RLS and PLMD. Polysomnography may also show pro-

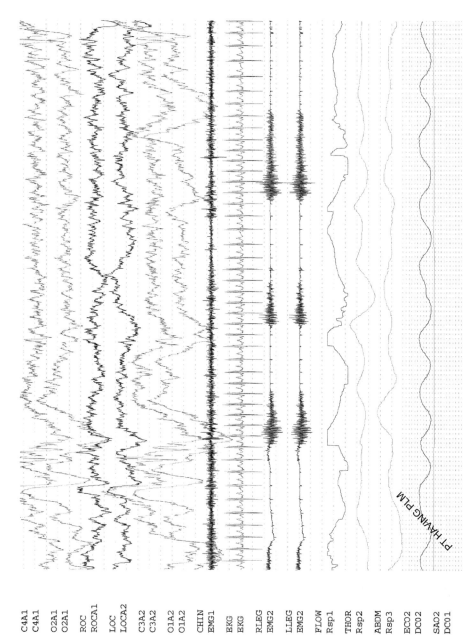

| C4A1 |
| C4A1 |
| O2A1 |
| O2A1 |
| ROC |
| ROCA1 |
| LOC |
| LOCA2 |
| C3A2 |
| C3A2 |
| O1A2 |
| O1A2 |
| CHIN |
| EMG1 |
| EKG |
| EKG |
| RLEG |
| EMG2 |
| LLEG |
| EMG2 |
| FLOW |
| Rsp1 |
| THOR |
| Rsp2 |
| ABDM |
| Rsp3 |
| ECO2 |
| DCO2 |
| SAO2 |
| DCO1 |

PT HAVING PLM

FIG. 14.1. Periodic limb movements.

longed sleep onset with frequent leg movements during awake time, at
bedtime, and possibly during nighttime awakenings.

- **PLMD:** PSG shows four or more consecutive leg movements lasting 0.5
  to 5 seconds, separated by 4- to 90-second intervals. To assess sleep disturbance, leg movements that are associated with an arousal (within 3 seconds of leg movement) or awakening are scored. An overall index per hour
  is provided, as is an index of limb movements associated with arousals. In
  both adults and children, a periodic limb movement (PLM) index >5 is
  considered pathologic (Fig. 14.1).
- **Labs:** Because of the association between RLS and iron deficiency anemia,
  especially low ferritin, a complete blood count and serum ferritin level
  (hemoglobin/hematocrit and indices may be normal) should be checked,
  particularly in children who may be at high risk for iron deficiency (toddlers, adolescent girls). In particular, a serum ferritin <50 is associated with
  RLS symptoms.

DIFFERENTIAL DIAGNOSIS

- **Prolonged sleep onset and nighttime awakenings** may result from insomnia,
  bedtime refusal, or general noncompliance (Chapters 6 and 17).
- **Excessive daytime sleepiness** can result from other sleep disorders, including
  obstructive sleep apnea, narcolepsy, idiopathic hypersomnolence, and insuffi-
  cient sleep.
- **Uncomfortable leg sensations** may be related to:
  - Nocturnal leg cramps
  - Sore muscles from overuse
  - Orthopedic conditions such as Osgood-Schlatter, chondromalacia patella
  - Chronic pain conditions such as juvenile rheumatoid arthritis
  - Peripheral neuropathy
  - Atopic dermatitis and pruritus
- **Sleep-related movements/restlessness** may be due to:
  - Sleep starts
  - Seizures
  - Apnea-related movements
  - Anxiety disorders

MANAGEMENT

When to Refer

If RLS or PLMD is suspected, referral to a sleep specialist for clinical diagnosis and/or overnight polysomnography is warranted.

Treatment

The decision of whether and when to treat RLS and/or PLMD depends on the level of severity (symptoms, sleep study results, and complications), sleep disruption, and daytime sequelae in a particular child or adolescent.

- **RLS.** If the symptoms of RLS result in prolonged sleep onset latency or severe complaints of leg discomfort, treatment is warranted.
- **PLMD.**
    - **PLM index > 10.** With moderate to severe disease, the treatment decision is usually straightforward.
    - **PLM index between 5 and 10.** For an index between 5 and 10, the decision to treat is based on the arousal index (if <5, no treatment may be warranted) and the presence or absence of other clinical sequelae (e.g., excessive daytime sleepiness, neurobehavioral complications).
    - **PLM index < 5.** For a PLM index between 1 and 5, usually no treatment is recommended.

Treatment Strategies

- **Sleep hygiene.** It is recommended that children with RLS maintain consistent bedtimes and bedtime routines, as well as obtain adequate nighttime sleep. Fatigue and drowsiness tend to exacerbate the symptoms of RLS. Furthermore, given that symptoms develop and/or increase with prolonged inactivity, it is best if children do not get into bed until ready to fall asleep. Thus, reading of bedtime stories and other such activities should occur in other places, such as in a nearby chair.
- **Additional nonpharmacologic treatments.** Moderate exercise up to a few hours before bedtime may suppress symptoms. Walking, stretching, massaging the affected area, and applying hot or cold packs may be helpful. Biofeedback and relaxation techniques may partially alleviate symptoms, as well as reduce stress. Keeping mentally occupied, especially during long periods of inactivity, should also be encouraged.
- **Substances to avoid.** Caffeine, alcohol, antihistamines, cold/sinus preparations, and antiemetics are known to exacerbate symptoms of RLS.
- **Iron and other supplements.** Iron supplements are warranted if serum ferritin levels are low. Supplementation with folate and vitamin B_{12} may be helpful in appropriate cases.
- **Medication.** No empirical studies have been conducted on the efficacy of specific medications for RLS/PLMD in children. The following recommendations are based on clinical experience. Governing principles in the use of medications for RLS in children are to use the lowest possible dose and to start at a minimal dose and titrate upward. The most commonly recommended medications are dopamine agonists and benzodiazepines, which generally improve

both the sensory and motor components. In adults, >90% of patients experience some relief of symptoms with medication.

The major medications used for RLS and PLMD in adults are listed below; dosages listed are usual ranges for adults. In choosing a medication to treat significant RLS/PLMD, consultation with a pediatric sleep specialist or neurologist is recommended.

- **Dopamine precursors:** Considered first line in adults; side effects include nausea, orthostatic hypotension, insomnia, daytime fatigue, and somnolence; augmentation in early evening (see below), morning rebound.
- *Levodopa with benserazide or carbidopa (Sinemet):* Regular or slow release; 100 to 125, 200 to 250 mg; at bedtime; may need additional dose during the night with regular preparation to avoid rebound periodic limb movements.
- **Dopamine agonists:** Used to treat both RLS and PLMD; side effects include nausea, orthostatic hypotension, insomnia, daytime fatigue, and somnolence; morning restlessness; tolerance may develop.
- *Pramipexole (Mirapex):* 0.125 to 1.0 mg at bedtime.
- *Pergolide (Permax):* 0.1 to 0.5 mg at bedtime.
- **Benzodiazepines:** Used to treat both RLS and PLMD; side effects include daytime sedation; may exacerbate obstructive sleep apnea symptoms, tolerance may develop.
- *Clonazepam (Klonopin):* 0.5 to 2.0 at bedtime.
- *Temazepam:* 15 to 30 mg at bedtime.
- *Nitrazepam:* 5 to 10 mg at bedtime.
- **Opiates:** Used to treat both RLS and PLMD; side effects include constipation and dependency.
- *Oxycodone (Percodan):* 5 mg at bedtime; may be repeated during the night if needed.
- *Propoxyphene (Darvon, Darvocet):* 200 mg at bedtime.
- *Codeine:* 15 to 60 mg at bedtime.
- **Anticonvulsants:** Used for RLS; side effects include daytime somnolence.
- *Carbamazepine (Tegretol):* 200 to 400 mg at bedtime.
- *Gabapentin (Neurontin):* 100 to 400 mg at bedtime.
- *Clonidine:* Used for RLS; side effects include hypotension; 0.05 to 0.2 mg at bedtime.

Many adult patients on medications, particularly those on dopaminergic agents, experience a phenomenon called augmentation. Augmentation is the worsening of RLS symptoms as a direct result of a specific therapeutic intervention; in many patients this takes the form of a shift in the timing of RLS symptoms to 2 or more hours earlier than the time symptoms are typically experienced. Augmentation generally occurs within 6 months of initiation of therapy and is usually responsive to a change in pharmacologic agent.

PROGNOSIS

No long-term studies have been conducted on the course of RLS or PLMD in children or adolescents. It is likely, however, that RLS and PLMD are chronic, lifelong disorders, although patients with milder disease may have long periods of remission. Cases of secondary RLS and PLMD generally remit without reoccurrence when the underlying condition is resolved.

Tips for Talking to Parents

- **Explain what RLS and PLMD are in simple terms,** including the associated sleep disruption.
- **Explain risk factors,** including anemia.
- **Review the daytime consequences,** as parents may not attribute hyperactivity or moodiness to a sleep problem.
- **Explain what to expect from the overnight sleep study.**
- **Review the results of the overnight sleep study.**
- **Discuss the risks and benefits of treatment options,** especially if medications are being considered.
- **Encourage any parent or family member with similar symptoms to be evaluated.**

See Appendix F10 for parent handout on restless legs syndrome and Appendix F11 on periodic limb movement disorder.

15

Narcolepsy

Narcolepsy is a neurologically based disorder that is characterized by uncontrollable and overwhelming daytime sleepiness. Narcolepsy is a lifelong disorder that often is first manifested in adolescence, and one that results in significant functional impairment and disability. The excessive daytime sleepiness involves repeated nap episodes ("sleep attacks") of short duration (10 to 20 minutes) throughout the day, following which the individual with narcolepsy usually feels temporarily refreshed. This sleepiness is often described as "irresistible" in that the child or adolescent is unable to stay awake even with effort, and occurs despite his or her obtaining a full night's sleep. Other symptoms that are part of the tetrad of symptoms of narcolepsy include cataplexy, hypnagogic hallucinations, and sleep paralysis.

Narcolepsy

Narcolepsy is a relatively rare chronic neurologic disorder that is accompanied by a significant degree of functional impairment. The hallmark of narcolepsy is excessive daytime sleepiness. Other symptoms that constitute the tetrad of symptoms are cataplexy, hypnagogic hallucinations, and sleep paralysis.

EPIDEMIOLOGY

- **Prevalence:** Narcolepsy is not a common disorder; its prevalence in the United States is reported to be between 3 and 16 per 10,000. However, the relative morbidity is increased by the significant level of functional impairment associated with narcolepsy and the frequent delay in diagnosis, in many cases for years after symptoms are first noted. It is estimated, for example, that as many as 200,000 Americans have narcolepsy but that fewer than 50,000 of those individuals have been diagnosed with the disorder.

- **Ethnicity:** Prevalence appears to vary with ethnicity:
  - 1/600 in Japan
  - 1/4,000 in North America and Europe
  - 1/500,000 in Israel
- **Gender:** Equal predominance in males and females.
- **Age:** Typically develops after puberty, with most individuals first reporting symptoms of narcolepsy between the ages of 15 and 30. Several studies have indicated that while as many as one third of adult patients report the onset of symptoms before age 15 years and another 16% before age 10 years, only about 4% of narcoleptics are diagnosed before the age of 15. The average time elapsed between onset of symptoms and diagnosis is 10 to 15 years.
- **Family history:** Positive family history of narcolepsy or excessive daytime sleepiness is found in a significant percentage of children with narcolepsy symptoms. It is estimated that 8% to 12% of individuals diagnosed with narcolepsy have a first-degree relative with the disease.

ETIOLOGY/RISK FACTORS

The pathophysiology of narcolepsy is based in the central nervous system and involves impaired sleep–wake regulation. The core symptoms of narcolepsy (cataplexy, sleep paralysis, and hypnagogic hallucinations) appear to represent a fundamental dysregulation of REM sleep. For example, cataplexy and sleep paralysis (described in the next section) seem to be the result of inappropriate inhibition of voluntary muscle tone during wakefulness, similar to what occurs during REM sleep. Hypnagogic hallucinations (also described below) occur in conjunction with REM sleep intrusion at sleep onset.

Recent discoveries in the past few years suggest an important role for the neurotransmitter orexin/hypocretin system, previously associated with feeding behavior and energy metabolism, in the neurophysiology of narcolepsy. Hypocretin is reduced or undetectable in many but not all patients with narcolepsy associated with cataplexy. It has been postulated that autoimmune mechanisms, possibly triggered by viral infections, in combination with environmental factors are involved.

The development of narcolepsy appears to involve both environmental and genetic factors. It is believed that familial narcolepsy is related to mutations in the genes synthesizing peptides in the hypocretin system or their receptors. Class II human leukocyte antigen (HLA) testing shows a strong genetic link, with more than 90% of European/Caucasian narcoleptics with cataplexy testing positive for HLA-DR2 (subtype DR15) and HLA-DQ1 (subtype DQB1-0602) antigens. In addition, children of narcoleptics have an increased risk for developing narcolepsy (1% risk, 40 times that of the general population). However, DR2-negative and DQ1-negative narcolepsy patients do exist, and DR2 has a 20% to 35% prevalence in the general population (>99% of those with this antigen do *not* have narcolepsy). Thus, the HLA-D gene is neither necessary nor sufficient to make the diagnosis. However, genetics do not account for all cases of narcolepsy as monozygotic twins have been found to be discordant for narcolepsy and there are cases in which no genetic predisposition has been found.

Although the majority of cases of narcolepsy are considered idiopathic, narcolepsy may also be associated with central nervous system trauma (following closed head injury); brain tumors (particularly in the third ventricle, posterior thalamic, and brainstem regions); and demyelinating processes, such as Niemann-Pick disease type C. Narcoleptic symptoms have been reported in association with Tourette syndrome, Turner syndrome, multiple sclerosis, and precocious puberty. The age of onset in these secondary or symptomatic narcolepsy cases tends to be lower (i.e., school aged).

PRESENTATION

- **Excessive daytime sleepiness** is the hallmark of narcolepsy. The irresistible urge to fall asleep occurs under conditions of low-level environmental stimulation, such as watching a movie or listening to a boring lecture, but also occurs in other situations, such as during a meal or while talking on the phone. In children, the naps tend to be longer and are also more likely to be described as "unrefreshing." Very brief (several seconds) attacks ("microsleeps") may also occur. The individual with narcolepsy is usually unaware of these microsleeps, which may be interpreted by observers as "daydreaming," inattentiveness/attention deficit-hyperactivity disorder (ADHD), or a possible manifestation of absence seizures.

The other symptoms that constitute the tetrad of narcolepsy symptoms are:

- **Cataplexy,** the abrupt loss of muscle tone provoked by a strong emotion. Cataplexy is the second most common symptom of narcolepsy, occurring in one study in as many as 80% of pediatric cases. The loss of muscle tone can range from localized sagging of the face, eyelids, or jaw to blurred vision to knee buckling to complete collapse. Laughter is the most common precipitator, but other emotions, such as surprise, anger, or sadness, can trigger cataplexy. During the episode, the individual maintains consciousness and memory is not impaired. The episode can last from seconds to minutes, with complete recovery. Episodes can range from occurring several times per day to a few times per year. Cataplexy is rarely the first symptom of narcolepsy, but it often develops within the first year of the onset of excessive daytime sleepiness.
- **Hypnagogic/hypnopompic hallucinations** involve vivid auditory or visual hallucinations, often described as "dreams." These occur during transitions between sleep and wakefulness, primarily at sleep onset (hypnagogic hallucination) and sleep offset (hypnopompic hallucination). Common hallucinations include faces and animals, often of a frightening or threatening nature. These hallucinations may be accompanied by sleep paralysis or occur independently and may also occur during daytime nap periods They are reported by approximately 50% to 70% of adult patients with narcolepsy. It should be noted, however, that hypnagogic/hypnopompic hallucinations are also occasionally experienced by normal individuals (in up to 10% of the population) without narcolepsy, especially in relation to sleep deprivation.

- **Sleep paralysis** is the inability to move or speak for a few seconds or minutes at sleep onset or offset. The paralysis ends spontaneously or after mild sensory stimulation (e.g., being shaken out of it). Sleep paralysis occurs in 40% to 65% of individuals with narcolepsy and may also accompany hypnagogic hallucinations. As with hypnagogic hallucinations, sleep paralysis is experienced by nonnarcoleptic individuals and therefore does not indicate the presence of narcolepsy.

Common Symptoms of Narcolepsy

- **Nighttime symptoms**
    Sleep disruption
    Hypnagogic hallucinations
    Sleep paralysis
- **Excessive daytime sleepiness**
    Falling asleep in school or at inappropriate times
    Short restorative naps
- **Daytime symptoms**
    Inattentiveness, poor concentration, distractibility
    Academic problems
    Automatic behaviors

Associated Features

- **Sleep disruption.** Nighttime sleep is often fragmented, and the child or adolescent may report nighttime awakenings. Furthermore, vivid dreams may be reported.
- **Naps.** Naps are usually short and restorative. In addition, many individuals with narcolepsy report dreaming during short naps.
- **Automatic behaviors.** Some individuals with narcolepsy report automatic behaviors that involve a semipurposeful activity of which there is no memory. These activities usually involve a repetitive or monotonous behavior, such as uttering words out of context or writing a page of nonsense in the midst of doing homework.
- **Impaired academic performance.** Given the propensity for falling asleep in school, many children and adolescents with narcolepsy experience problems with academic performance. In addition, children and adolescents with narcolepsy are often labeled as lazy, inattentive, and difficult.

The Great Masquerader

The symptoms of narcolepsy (e.g., excessive daytime sleepiness, cataplexy) are frequently misdiagnosed, particularly in children and adolescents, as psychiatric or behavioral disorders, including ADHD, depression, conversion reaction, and even psychosis.

TABLE 15.1. *Diagnostic criteria: narcolepsy (347)*

Diagnostic Criteria:
A. A complaint of excessive sleepiness or sudden muscle weakness
B. Recurrent daytime naps or lapses into sleep that occur almost daily for at least 3 months
C. Sudden bilateral loss of postural muscle tone in association with intense emotion (cataplexy)
D. Associated features include:
   1. Sleep paralysis
   2. Hypnagogic hallucinations
   3. Automatic behaviors
   4. Disrupted major sleep episode
E. Polysomnography demonstrates one or more of the following:
   1. Sleep latency less than 10 minutes
   2. REM sleep latency less than 20 minutes
   3. An MSLT that demonstrates a mean sleep latency of less than 5 minutes
   4. Two or more sleep-onset REM periods (on MSLT)
F. Human leukocyte antigen typing demonstrates DR2 positivity
G. Absence of any medical or psychiatric disorder that could account for the symptoms
H. Other sleep disorders may be present, but are not the primary cause of the symptoms

Minimal criteria: B plus C, or A plus D plus E plus G.
MSLT, multiple sleep latency time; REM, rapid eye movement.
Used with permission from American Acacemy of Sleep Medicine. *The international classification of sleep disorders, revised: diagnostic and coding manual.* Westchester, IL: AASM, 1997: 42–43.

Diagnostic Criteria

See Table 15.1.

EVALUATION

- **Medical history:** A thorough medical history should include evaluation of other possible causes of excessive daytime sleepiness, such as obstructive sleep apnea, restless legs syndrome, periodic limb movement disorder, psychiatric disorders, neurologic conditions, use of prescription and nonprescription medications, and alcohol and drug use. Because narcolepsy may be secondary to underlying medical conditions (e.g., head injury, central nervous system tumors, demyelinating disorders), a thorough history should include screening for these concerns. There have been a number of case reports that have documented an association between narcolepsy and obesity and hyperphagia in children; the significance of this relationship is currently unknown but raises some intriguing questions about the role of the hypocretin system.
- **Developmental/school history:** Generally normal, although children with secondary narcolepsy associated with underlying neurologic disorders such as Niemann-Pick disease type C will obviously have developmental delays. There may be a history suggestive of attentional problems; older children and adolescents with narcolepsy frequently have a history of significant academic concerns.
- **Family history:** Positive in first-degree relatives in an estimated 10% of cases, although other studies have found a lower percentage (3% to 5%). Up to 40%

of individuals may have a family member with a history of excessive daytime sleepiness.

- **Behavioral assessment:** May indicate attention problems, mood issues, and behavioral concerns such as hyperactivity and poor impulse control. Because of the functional impairment associated with the excessive daytime sleepiness, older children and adolescents with undiagnosed narcolepsy may have significant social problems as well. There have been case reports of individuals with daytime hypnagogic/hypnopompic hallucinations who have been misdiagnosed with psychosis.
- **Physical examination:** In the majority of cases, the physical examination is completely normal. An abnormal neurologic examination suggests the possibility of secondary narcolepsy and requires appropriate additional diagnostic evaluation (e.g., neuroimaging). Excessive daytime sleepiness in the office setting may be noted.
- **Diagnostic tests**
  - **Overnight sleep study (polysomnography) and MSLT.** Overnight polysomnography and multiple sleep latency test (MSLT) are mandatory components of the evaluation of a patient with suspected narcolepsy. The MSLT is a series of four scheduled naps of 20 minutes duration on the day following polysomnography that objectively quantifies daytime sleepiness and assesses the presence of sleep onset REM periods, which are a marker for narcolepsy. Prior to polysomnography, the child or adolescent should be withdrawn from any medications that affect the central nervous system and told to follow a regular sleep schedule for at least 2 weeks. In children and adolescents, it should be noted that it may take several polysomnographic studies over a period of 6 months to several years to make a definitive diagnosis.
    - *Polysomnography diagnostic criteria (adult criteria):*
      - Sleep latency < 10 minutes
      - REM sleep latency < 20 minutes
    - *MSLT diagnostic criteria (adult criteria):*
      - MSLT mean sleep latency < 5 minutes
      - Two or more sleep onset REM periods during the MSLT
  - **Neuroimaging (magnetic resonance imaging)** is indicated with sudden onset of significant sleepiness, recent head injury, or abnormal neurologic examination.

DIFFERENTIAL DIAGNOSIS

- **Chronic sleep deprivation** and erratic sleep–wake schedules can produce significant daytime sleepiness; however, maintenance of an appropriate sleep schedule will alleviate daytime symptoms.
- **Prolonged sleep need** may lead to daytime sleepiness if the sleep schedule does not provide adequate sleep. Individuals with narcolepsy typically do not sleep more hours than average at night and awaken refreshed in the morning.

TABLE 15.2. *Differential diagnosis for narcolepsy and idiopathic hypersomnia*

Narcolepsy	Idiopathic hypersomnia
Comparison of Symptoms	
Disrupted nocturnal sleep	Prolonged or deep sleep
Naps are frequent and restorative	Naps are not restorative
Cataplexy	No cataplexy
Never remits	Reports of remission
Other associated symptoms	May follow viral infection or head trauma
Diagnostic Criteria	
PSG:	PSG:
• Short sleep latency	• Short sleep latency
• Short REM sleep latency	• Normal REM latency
• Normal sleep period	• Prolonged sleep period
MSLT:	MSLT:
• Sleep latency <5 min	• Sleep latency <10 min
• ≥2 Sleep onset REM periods	• <2 Sleep onset REM periods

MSLT, multiple sleep latency test; PSG, polysomnogram; REM, rapid eye movement.

- **Underlying sleep disrupters,** including obstructive sleep apnea (see Chapter 13), restless legs syndrome (see Chapter 14), and periodic limb movement disorder (see Chapter 14), can result in excessive daytime sleepiness.
- **Idiopathic hypersomnia** symptoms overlap considerably those of narcolepsy. All symptoms occur in both disorders, except for cataplexy. In addition, the presence of DQ1 antigen is increased in idiopathic hypersomnia. See Table 15.2 for a comparison of symptoms and diagnostic criteria.
- **Kleine-Levin syndrome** involves episodic hypersomnolence (12 hours to 4 weeks), as well as abnormal behaviors (overeating and hypersexuality). Kleine-Levin is more common in boys, and the usual onset is during adolescence.
- **Psychiatric disorders depression** should be considered in children and adolescents who present with significant sleepiness and associated neurobehavioral symptoms. Conversion reactions may mimic cataplectic attacks. However, it should be noted that the same pharmacologic agents that are used for particular psychiatric conditions (stimulants for ADHD, tricyclic antidepressants for depression) also improve symptoms of narcolepsy. Therefore, treatment response to these agents should not be used to differentiate psychiatric disorders from narcolepsy.
- **Other neurologic causes** of sleepiness can result in daytime sleepiness, such as posttraumatic hypersomnia, medications, and alcohol or drug use.

MANAGEMENT

When to Refer

Children or adolescents with suspected narcolepsy should be referred to a sleep specialist or pediatric neurologist for diagnosis and management. Any pharmacologic treatment should be done in consultation with one of these specialists.

Treatment

Narcolepsy cannot be cured, but its symptoms can usually be controlled so that a child or adolescent with narcolepsy can lead a normal life. Each treatment plan usually involves education, behavioral changes, and medication.

- **Patient and family education.** Narcolepsy can be a devastating disorder without appropriate education. Daytime sleepiness may be mistaken for laziness, boredom, or lack of ability. The experiences of cataplexy and dreaming during wakefulness may be wrongly seen as a psychiatric problem. Education should not only include all family members, but also teachers and friends.
- **Sleep hygiene.** Positive sleep habits are essential for children and adolescents with narcolepsy (see Appendices F15 and F16), as is obtaining adequate nighttime sleep.
- **Napping.** Prescribed short naps once or twice a day can help control the daytime sleepiness, although they are seldom sufficient as a primary therapy.
- **Behavioral changes.** Lifestyle changes can provide substantial improvement of symptoms.
  - A strict sleep–wake schedule that ensures adequate sleep is essential.
  - Increased physical activity, with avoidance of boring or repetitive tasks, can be helpful.
  - Avoidance of activities, such as driving, swimming, or cooking, that can be dangerous is essential, except during times when the child or adolescent is alert. All adolescents with narcolepsy must be well controlled prior to receiving permission to drive.
- **Medications.** Medications are often prescribed to control the excessive daytime sleepiness. The goal should be to allow the fullest possible return of normal functioning in school, at home, and in social situations. Medication may also be used to control the REM-associated phenomena, such as cataplexy, hypnagogic hallucinations, and sleep paralysis, when these are clinically significant and affect the patient's quality of life. These agents are often used in combination to treat the individual's symptom constellation. As there is relatively little long-term experience with many of these medications in children and adolescents, most of the information is based on adult studies.

Stimulant medications for excessive daytime sleepiness:
  - **Methylphenidate (Ritalin):** safe and generally well tolerated. *Suggested prepubertal child dose:* 5 to 10 mg BID/TID. Adolescent dose: 10 to 20 mg BID/TID; consider single long-acting preparation (Concerta) in morning.
  - **Dextroamphetamine (Dexedrine):** safe and generally well tolerated; more likely to result in development of tolerance. *Suggested prepubertal child dose:* 2.5 to 5 mg BID/TID or 5 to 10 mg spansule BID. Adolescent

dose: 15 mg spansule BID; consider single long-acting. preparation (Adderall XR) in morning. Combinations of long-acting (Metadate, Concerta, Adderall) and short-acting forms of stimulants may be necessary to achieve adequate coverage.

- **Pemoline (Cylert);** rarely used because of rare reports of potentially lethal liver toxicity
- **Modafinil (Provigil);** classified as "somnolytic" rather than "stimulant" medication, α_1-adrenergic system action; lower risk for cardiovascular and psychiatric side effects than stimulants; no associated mood changes or dependence potential; side effects include headaches, anxiety, depression, nausea, diarrhea, decreased appetite, and dry mouth; may cause eosinophilia; may interact with anticonvulsants. *Suggested prepubertal child dose:* start with 100 mg in morning for 5 days; add second noontime 100-mg dose as needed. *Adolescent dose:* start with 100 mg in morning for 5 days, add additional 100 mg in morning as needed, add noontime 100-mg dose as needed. Maximal adult dose 400 mg; may combine with "traditional" stimulants (e.g., methylphenidate).

Failure to respond to psychostimulants or modafinil prescribed at an adequate dosage range should prompt a reevaluation for other possible causes of or contributory factors for excessive daytime sleepiness.

REM suppressants for cataplexy, hypnagogic hallucinations, sleep paralysis:
- **Tricyclic antidepressants, such as protriptyline (Vivactil), imipramine (Tofranil), clomipramine (Anafranil):** Start at lower than usual antidepressant doses and titrate up; use more sedating medication at bedtime and more alerting medication for daytime; increase in muscle tone associated with use may precipitate periodic limb movements during sleep; abrupt discontinuation may cause rebound cataplexy, sleep paralysis, and hypnogogic hallucinations. *Suggested prepubertal child doses:* clomipramine 25 to 50 mg at bedtime. *Adolescent dose:* clomipramine 50 mg at bedtime.
- **Other antidepressants (selective serotonin reuptake inhibitors, or SSRIs),** such as *fluoxetine (Prozac), venlafaxine (Effexor):* typically prescribed at usual antidepressant doses; may be less effective than tricyclics but with fewer side effects. *Suggested prepubertal child dose:* fluoxetine 10 to 20 mg in morning or venlafaxine 75 to 150 mg in morning. *Adolescent dose:* fluoxetine 10 to 40 mg in morning or venlafaxine 75 to 150 mg in morning (Table 15.3)

PROGNOSIS

Narcolepsy is a chronic, lifelong disorder that will always require management. The goal of treatment is adaptation and improved quality of life.

TABLE 15.3. *Pharmacological treatment of narcolepsy in children and adolescents*

Prepubertal children	Pubertal children
General Measures	**General Measures**
Contact school to alert teachers	Contact school to alert teachers
Nap at lunch time	Emphasize need for regular nocturnal sleep
Nap at 4 or 5 PM	schedule
	Try to obtain 9 hr of nocturnal sleep
	Nap at lunch time and 4 or 5 PM
Medication for Sleepiness	**Medication for Sleepiness**
Methylphenidate 5 mg (2–4) tablets	Methylphenidate 5 mg (2–6 tablets[a]) or 20 mg
	SR in the morning (on empty stomach)
Modafinil 100–200 mg[b]	Modafinil[b] 100–400 mg
Medication for Cataplexy[c]	**Medication for Cataplexy**[c]
Clomipramine 25–50 mg at bedtime	Clomipramine 50 mg at bedtime
Fluoxetine 10–20 mg in the morning	Fluoxetine 10–40 mg in the morning
Venlafaxine 75–150 mg (in the morning)	Venlafaxine 75–150 mg (in the morning)

SR, sustained-release tablet.

[a]Usually 10 mg when waking up on an empty stomach, 5 mg around lunchtime, and 5 mg at 3 PM.

[b]Modafinil is started at 100 mg in the morning for 5 days, and a second dose of 100 mg is then added at lunchtime, if needed. This is usually sufficient in prepubertal children. Pubertal children may require a further increase (after 5 days) to an additional 100 mg in the morning, and, if still needed later, another 100 mg at noon.

[c]The use of antidepressants for cataplexy is not Food and Drug Administration (FDA) approved. No medications have specifically received approval by the FDA for use in narcolepsy patients younger than 16 years.

From Guilleminault C, Anagnos A. Narcolepsy. In: Kryger MH, Roth T, Dement WC, eds. *Principles and practice of sleep medicine.* Philadelphia: WB Saunders, 2002.

Tips for Talking to Parents

- **Explain what narcolepsy is** in simple terms, including the lack of control over excessive daytime sleepiness, as well as the other tetrad of symptoms.
- **Explain the genetic and neurological basis** of narcolepsy.
- **Review the daytime consequences of narcolepsy.** Parents may not attribute daytime sleepiness, academic problems, and apparent inattention, for example, to a sleep problem.
- **Explain what to expect from the overnight sleep study and multiple sleep latency test.**
- **Review the results of the overnight sleep study.** In interpreting the study's implications, it is important to ask the child or adolescent if his/her usual level of daytime sleepiness was experienced the day of testing.
- **Discuss the risks and benefits of treatment options,** including lifestyle changes and medication choices.
- **Encourage any parent or other family member who experiences excessive daytime sleepiness** to be evaluated for narcolepsy.

See Appendix F12 for parent handout on narcolepsy.

16

Delayed Sleep Phase Syndrome

Delayed sleep phase syndrome (DSPS), a circadian rhythm disorder, involves a significant, persistent, and intractable phase shift in sleep–wake schedule (later bedtime and waketime) that conflicts with the individual's school, work, and/or lifestyle demands. It is the timing rather than the quality of sleep per se that is problematic. Delayed sleep phase syndrome may occur at any age, but is most common in adolescents and young adults. Individuals with delayed sleep phase syndrome often start out as "night owls"; that is, they have an underlying predisposition or circadian preference for staying up late at night and sleeping late in the morning, especially on weekends, holidays, and summer vacations. The typical sleep–wake pattern in delayed sleep phase syndrome is a consistently preferred bedtime/sleep onset time after midnight, and waketime after 10 AM, 7 days a week.

Delayed Sleep Phase Syndrome

Delayed sleep phase syndrome, a circadian rhythm disorder, involves a significant, persistent, and intractable shift in sleep–wake schedules that interferes with environmental demands, usually resulting in significant academic and behavior problems.

Adolescents with delayed sleep phase syndrome may complain of sleep onset insomnia and extreme difficulty waking in the morning, even for desired activities. In order to cope, many adolescents with delayed sleep phase syndrome take lengthy afternoon naps or catch up by extending sleep on weekends and days off. With delayed sleep phase syndrome, even highly motivated adolescents are unable to shift their sleep back to an earlier time without assistance.

EPIDEMIOLOGY

- **Prevalence.** Studies indicate that delayed sleep phase syndrome affects approximately 5% to 10% of adolescents.
- **Age of onset.** Onset is typically during adolescence, when an underlying circadian preference for late bedtime/waketime ("eveningness") may become exaggerated. Younger children with a marked phase delay may also develop delayed sleep phase syndrome.
- **Gender.** There is some evidence to suggest a male predominance in younger populations.

ETIOLOGY/RISK FACTORS

It appears that delayed sleep phase syndrome involves an intrinsic abnormality in the circadian oscillators that govern the timing of the sleep period. Nocturnal melatonin secretion appears to be delayed in these individuals. Evidence supporting a primarily neurobiological substrate for this disorder also includes persistence of the disorder in the face of significant academic and social consequences, high rates of relapse following successful intervention, and some evidence supporting a genetic component. One of the major risk factors for the development of delayed sleep phase syndrome is an intrinsic evening preference that is exacerbated after puberty when there is a normal physiologic delay in shift by approximately 2 hours. These physiologic changes often coincide with changes in schedule demands (e.g., earlier school start times in high school), resulting in chronic insufficient sleep.

In addition, those children or adolescents experiencing difficulties in school or school refusal may present with a preferred or "motivated" phase delay—risk factors that favor persistence of symptoms and make the disorder more difficult to treat. The relationship between psychiatric disorders and delayed sleep phase syndrome is a complex one; delayed sleep phase syndrome may result in symptoms of depression, and the insomnia associated with primary depression may mimic delayed sleep phase syndrome.

PRESENTATION

- **Sleep onset** at a consistently late time, usually after midnight in adolescents.
- **Minimal difficulty with sleep maintenance,** with infrequent nighttime awakenings.
- **Significant difficulty waking** at the required time (e.g., waking for school) and decreased alertness in the morning.
- **Persistent difficulty going to sleep at an earlier time** than the preferred bedtime. Although, with effort, the individual with delayed sleep phase syndrome may temporarily achieve sleep onset at an earlier time, there is a natural tendency to "drift" to the later preferred bedtime.

- **Complaints of "insomnia,"** if the adolescent attempts to go to sleep at an earlier time; however, no sleep onset insomnia is experienced if bedtime coincides with the preferred sleep onset time (e.g., on weekends, school vacations).
- **Daytime sleepiness** (e.g., napping, dozing off, mood changes, inattentiveness), in addition to difficulty waking in the morning, may be experienced throughout the day due to chronic insufficient sleep.

Associated Features

- **Bedtime resistance** and delayed sleep onset in younger children. Children with an evening preference may have difficulty falling asleep at an age-appropriate bedtime, leading to protests, excuses, and oppositional behavior.
- **Evening or night preference,** with optimal functioning ("second wind") during the late afternoon, evening, and night hours.
- **Weekend "oversleep"** until late morning/early afternoon in an attempt to make up for weekday insufficient sleep. Extended sleep periods are often seen during vacations as well, especially in the first few days of the vacation.
- **Poor school performance,** as adolescents with delayed sleep phase syndrome are often chronically sleep deprived and thus, even when highly motivated, may perform poorly in school.
- **School tardiness and frequent absenteeism** is often present. The sleep problem may lead to a downward spiral of missed school due to the frequent tardiness and absences, resulting in academic failure and subsequently in more school avoidance. In severe cases, the child or adolescent may "give up" going to school altogether.

Diagnostic Criteria

See Table 16.1.

EVALUATION

- **Medical history:** Generally benign.
- **Developmental/school history:** Parents often note that these children are often lifelong "night owls." Questions regarding morningness–eveningness ("owl–lark") preferences may reveal a patterns of alertness and sleepiness during the day that is delayed relative to normal circadian peaks and troughs. Questions about "feel best" times for going to bed, morning waking, and performing various tasks (e.g., taking tests, playing a sport) may be helpful in confirming a pattern of delayed circadian rhythms. Furthermore, academic problems are common and usually a result of the sleep disorder. When academic concerns predate the sleep problem, there may be an element of school avoidance compounding the situation.

- **Family history:** May reveal other family members with a marked evening circadian preference.
- **Behavioral assessment:** It is extremely important to assess for possible substance use and psychiatric issues, including depression, anxiety disorders, school refusal, and school phobia.
- **Physical exam:** Generally benign.
- **Diagnostic tests:**
  - **Sleep diaries.** Recording of sleep–wake patterns is a very important component of the evaluation for delayed sleep phase syndrome and will often graphically demonstrate the sleep phase delay and consistent fall-asleep/wake-up times.
  - **Polysomnography.** In general, overnight sleep studies are not indicated unless there is a concern regarding possible underlying sleep-disrupting factors.

TABLE 16.1. *Diagnostic criteria: Delayed Sleep-Phase Syndrome (780.55)*

A. The patient has a complaint of an inability to fall asleep at the desired clock time, an inability to awaken spontaneously at the desired time of awakening, or excessive sleepiness.
B. There is a phase delay of the major sleep episode in relation to the desired time for sleep.
C. The symptoms are present for at least one month.
D. When not required to maintain a strict sleep schedule (e.g., vacation time), patients will exhibit all of the following:
  1. Have a habitual sleep period that is sound and of normal quality and duration
  2. Awaken spontaneously
  3. Maintain sleep entrainment to a 24-hr sleep–wake pattern at a delayed phase
E. Sleep–wake logs that are maintained daily for a period of at least 2 weeks must demonstrate evidence of a delay in the timing of the habitual sleep period.
F. One of the following laboratory methods must demonstrate a delay in the timing of the habitual sleep period:
  1. Twenty-four-hour polysomnographic monitoring (or by means of two consecutive nights of polysomnography and an intervening multiple sleep latency test)
  2. Continuous temperature monitoring showing that the time of the absolute temperature nadir is delayed into the second half of the habitual (delayed) sleep episode
G. The symptoms do not meet the criteria for any other sleep disorder causing inability to initiate sleep or excessive sleepiness.

Minimal criteria: A plus B plus C plus D plus E.
Used with permission from American Academy of Sleep Medicine. *The international classification of sleep disorders, revised: diagnostic and coding manual.* Westchester, IL: AASM, 1997: 132–133.

Morningness–Eveningness Preference

Sample questions to assess morningness or eveningness circadian preference:

1. If you were entirely free to plan your evening and had no commitments the next day, at what time would you choose to go to bed?
   1. 8:00–9:00 PM
   2. 9:00–10:15 PM
   3. 10:15 PM–12:30 AM
   4. 12:30–1:45 AM
   5. 1:45–3:00 AM
2. For some reason you have gone to bed several hours later than normal, but there is no need to get up at a particular time the next morning. Which of the following is most likely to occur?
   1. Will wake up at the usual time and not fall asleep again
   2. Will wake up at the usual time and doze thereafter
   3. Will wake up at the usual time but will fall asleep again
   4. Will not wake up until later than usual
3. You have to take a 2-hour test. If you were entirely free to choose, in which of the following periods would you prefer to take the test?
   1. 8:00–10:00 AM
   2. 11:00 AM–1:30 PM
   3. 3:00–5:00 PM
   4. 7:00–9:00 PM
4. If you had no commitments the next day and were entirely free to plan your own day, what time would you get up?
   1. 5:00–6:30 AM
   2. 6:30–7:45 AM
   3. 7:45–9:45 AM
   4. 9:45–11:00 AM
   5. 11:00 AM–12:00 PM

Adapted from Horne JA, Ostberg O. A self assessment questionnaire to determine morningness–eveningness in human circadian rhythms. *Int J Chronobiol* 1976;4:97–110.

DIFFERENTIAL DIAGNOSIS

- **Insomnia.** Difficulties falling asleep at night may be the result of psychophysiologic or "learned" insomnia (see Chapter 17). One clear differentiating factor between the two is that children and adolescents with delayed sleep phase syndrome have few or no difficulties falling asleep if they go to bed at their preferred sleep onset time. However, individuals with insomnia experience difficulties falling asleep no matter what time they go to bed and do not exhibit a consistent fall-asleep time.

- **Restless legs syndrome.** Symptoms of restless legs syndrome (e.g., uncomfortable sensations in the legs at bedtime relieved by movement; see Chapter 14) often present with delayed sleep onset.
- **Poor sleep hygiene,** including maintenance of an erratic sleep schedule and use of caffeine or other substances, may result in complaints of difficulty falling asleep. It should be noted that individuals with delayed sleep phase syndrome might also develop sleep habits that are ultimately counterproductive (such as lying in bed awake for long periods) in an attempt to "fix" their sleep problem. These secondary poor sleep habits must also be addressed in treatment programs. However, individuals with delayed sleep phase syndrome will still have delayed sleep onset, even after the establishment of an appropriate sleep schedule and the institution of appropriate sleep habits.
- **Circadian preference.** Although a preference for evening hours ("night owl") is a risk factor for delayed sleep phase syndrome, eveningness does not have the same intractable quality and persistence, and does not result in significantly compromised functioning.
- **Lifestyle issues** (e.g., socializing, late-night television viewing). These can result in delayed sleep times, difficulty awakening in the morning, and insufficient sleep.
- **School avoidance or refusal.** Adolescents with primary school avoidance, such as that resulting from an anxiety disorder or related to a learning disability and academic failure, may have a late bedtime and appear difficult to awaken in the morning. In this situation, the sleep schedule is not intractable, and a more appropriate sleep schedule may be maintained on weekends and holidays.
- **Psychiatric disorders** (e.g., depression, bipolar disorder, anxiety disorders). Many psychiatric conditions are associated with difficulty falling asleep, but the set sleep–wake schedule pattern that is characteristic of delayed sleep phase syndrome is not usually present in these situations, and the sleep disturbance will covary with the psychiatric symptoms.

MANAGEMENT

When to Refer

Children or adolescents with delayed sleep phase syndrome who also demonstrate symptoms of other underlying sleep disrupters (e.g., obstructive sleep apnea) should be referred to a sleep specialist. Where there are concerns regarding school refusal, depression, or other psychological issues, referral to a mental health specialist is warranted. Treatment programs involving chronotherapy, light therapy, and melatonin are often best accomplished in consultation with a sleep specialist.

Treatment

The goal in the treatment of delayed sleep phase syndrome is basically twofold: first, shifting the sleep–wake schedule to an earlier time, and second, maintaining the new schedule. The choice of a target bedtime and waketime should be discussed with the patient and family in the context of balancing the primary goal of adequate sleep with lifestyle considerations. The initial treatment phase is generally more intense and requires strict adherence to the treatment protocol; the maintenance phase is necessary because of the natural tendency of these individuals to gradually shift to a later bedtime and waketime. Successful treatment requires a motivated patient and family, a coordinated approach that involves changes in sleep habits, and may include chronotherapy, medication, and/or bright-light therapy

---

Motivation: Key to Successful Treatment

A highly motivated adolescent is required, as achieving success in realigning an adolescent's sleep schedule and maintaining the change can be difficult. Thus, issues such as the motivation of the child/adolescent, the resources of the family, and the existence of any psychiatric or substance abuse problems must first be addressed before success can be expected. Sufficient motivation for (and barriers to) instituting change must be explored. Similar to many other behavioral interventions, a well-developed plan is essential to achieve success. Behavioral contracts are often necessary, and psychological and family issues may need to be addressed if resistance to change is encountered, as is frequently the case.

Shifting the circadian rhythm: Phase advancement and phase delay (chronotherapy). Treatment for delayed sleep phase syndrome involves shifting the circadian sleep—wake rhythm so that sleep and morning waking occurs at the desired time. There are two primary strategies to accomplish this shift:
- **Phase advancement.** Phase advancement is used when the difference between the current later sleep onset time and the target earlier sleep onset time is less than 3 hours. Bedtimes and waketimes are shifted earlier by approximately 15 minutes per day, beginning with the time that the adolescent usually falls asleep without difficulty. Thus, if the patient is not falling asleep until 1:30 AM, then the first night bedtime is set for 1:15, then 1:00, and so on. The shift is done gradually to increase the likelihood that the patient will be able to fall asleep relatively quickly at the successively earlier bedtimes, which avoids prolonged periods of lying awake in bed. The pace (shifting the bedtime earlier every day versus every 2 or 3 days) and the

time increment of the shift (advancing by 5 minutes versus 15 or 30 minutes) is somewhat dependent on the chronicity of the delayed sleep phase problem (the longer the duration, the more gradual the process needed), the patient's ongoing response to treatment, and how quickly the shift to the target bedtime/waketime must be accomplished. An additional sleep scheduling strategy that is often helpful is sleep restriction. This process involves setting the morning waketime at the target earlier waketime right at the beginning of treatment while more gradually advancing the bedtime over several weeks. Sleep restriction assists in accomplishing the phase shift by causing relative sleep deprivation during the initial period of treatment, thus increasing the likelihood that the patient will be ready to fall asleep at the earlier bedtime.

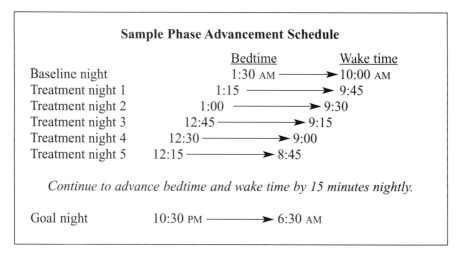

Sample Phase Advancement Schedule

	Bedtime	Wake time
Baseline night	1:30 AM ────→	10:00 AM
Treatment night 1	1:15 ────→	9:45
Treatment night 2	1:00 ────→	9:30
Treatment night 3	12:45 ────→	9:15
Treatment night 4	12:30 ────→	9:00
Treatment night 5	12:15 ────→	8:45

Continue to advance bedtime and wake time by 15 minutes nightly.

| Goal night | 10:30 PM ────→ | 6:30 AM |

- **Phase delay (chronotherapy).** Phase delay is used for more severely delayed sleep phase cases (e.g., shift is greater than 3 hours) and involves delaying bedtime and waketime by 2 to 3 hours daily. Thus, if an adolescent usually goes to bed at 4:00 AM, on the first day of intervention bedtime is scheduled for 7:00 AM, the second day 10:00 AM, and so on until the desired time is achieved. Adolescents are often compliant during the first phase of this treatment because of the perception that they are being "allowed" to stay up later each day. Since the patient is usually sleepy by the successively later scheduled sleep times, delayed sleep onset is not a problem; however, the patient may have difficulty remaining awake for an additional 2 to 3 hours each day and may need family support and supervision to accomplish this. Chronotherapy requires considerable motivation and commitment on the adolescent's part as the treatment phase is quite disruptive. If possible, chronotherapy should be timed to coincide with a school vacation to avoid missing school during the period of daytime sleep.

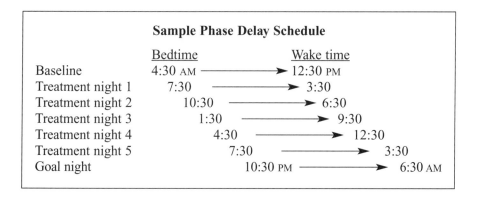

Sleep hygiene
 • **Sleep habits.** The patient's sleep habits should be reviewed and reorganized if necessary, with an emphasis on the development of positive sleep routines and avoidance of caffeine. Secondary poor sleep habits, such as lying in bed awake for long periods, also need to be addressed (see Appendices F15 and F16).
 • **Maintain schedule.** Napping must be avoided to help consolidate sleep. In addition, the patient must maintain a consistent sleep schedule both on weekdays and weekends, even after the initial treatment phase is completed.

Additional treatment strategies
 • **Pharmacotherapy.** Although there are some potential risks (see Chapter 19), some authors have reported that oral melatonin supplementation (1 to 5 mg) taken about an hour before the prescribed bedtime can be beneficial in inducing sleepiness (mildly sedating), as well as shifting the sleep–wake phase.
 • **Bright light.** Exposure to bright light upon waking is beneficial to help reset the sleep–wake rhythm. In uncomplicated or mild cases, light exposure can consist of eating breakfast in a sunny area of the home, spending time outdoors first thing in the morning, and avoiding sunglasses in the morning hours. In more difficult cases, morning exposure to 20 to 30 minutes of bright light (10,000 lux) provided by a specially designed light box unit upon awakening can be beneficial. Commercially produced light boxes or lamps are portable units, which combine high-output (2,500 to 10,000 lux) fluorescent tubes with reflectors, and can be obtained online at such sites as *www.apollolight.com, www.lighttherapyproducts.com*, and *www. alaskanorthernlights.com*. Light exposure therapy should be continued for at least 2 to 4 weeks. Patients may also benefit from avoiding exposure to bright light in the early evening during the intense treatment phase in order to help reset the circadian clock. Dark glasses may be worn during exposure to sunlight late in the day. Patients may also benefit from avoiding exposure to bright light in the early evening.

Tips for Bright Light Exposure Therapy

- As each manufacturer has different specifications, it is important to read instructions carefully for the individual light box or lamp unit.
- The UV filter (if needed) should be in place before use.
- The patient should not look directly at the light but make sure the light shines on the eyes; no sunglasses should be worn.
- Distance from the light box unit and head position determines the light intensity delivered. If engaging in other activities (reading, eating) while using the light box, the light should be positioned about 16 to 20 inches from the patient, at head or chest level.
- Some patients experience eye/skin irritation (especially patients with fair skin, light eye color), queasiness, and headaches with use of a light box. If this occurs, increasing the distance of the light box and decreasing the exposure time before gradually increasing it may help.
- Some antibiotics and acne/retinoic acid creams may increase light sensitivity.

- **Additional issues**
  - **Maintenance phase.** Treatment for delayed sleep phase syndrome usually involves an intense treatment phase, during which there can be no deviation from the prescribed schedule. Following this phase, there will be a protracted maintenance phase, which is also quite difficult. Many find this phase to be the more difficult aspect of treatment. All it takes is one weekend or vacation in which old habits are resumed to undo all achievements. Once the new schedule is firmly entrenched an occasional late night is permitted, but the adolescent should not be allowed to sleep more than 1 or 2 hours later than his or her usual weekday waketime.
  - **Additional issues.** Other issues must be addressed if warranted, such as school refusal and other psychiatric problems (e.g., depression, substance use).

PROGNOSIS

Delayed sleep phase syndrome is often a chronic disorder but with high motivation can be changed. However, a high rate of relapse following initial treatment success is common.

Tips for Talking to Parents

- **Describe delayed sleep phase syndrome,** emphasizing the intractable nature of the circadian clock with this disorder.
- **Discuss treatment options,** including phase advancement or phase delay.
- **Encourage parents to have the child or adolescent take responsibility for the sleep schedule.**
- **Explain the role of sleep hygiene in treatment success.**
- **Discuss issues of sleep schedule maintenance** following the shift in the circadian rhythm.

See Appendix F13 for parent handout on delayed sleep phase syndrome.

17

Insomnia

Insomnia is broadly defined as significant subjective difficulty initiating and/or maintaining sleep and/or early morning awakening, and represents a more global sleep symptom complex. Insomnia is one of the most common sleep complaints in adults, but parents (as well as children and adolescents themselves) are much less likely to present with "insomnia" as the chief concern. The complaint of insomnia can be short term and transient, usually related to a stressful event, or can be long term and chronic.

Because insomnia is a *symptom* rather than a sleep disorder, it can be associated with a variety of sleep problems or medical issues. When the insomnia is not secondary to another sleep disturbance, or to a psychiatric or medical problem, it is referred to as **psychophysiologic insomnia** (according to the *International Classification of Sleep Disorders*) or **primary insomnia** (according to the *Diagnostic and Statistical Manual*, 4th ed.). It is sometimes also called "learned insomnia" or "behavioral insomnia." It becomes a disorder rather than a symptom when accompanied by learned sleep-preventing associations and physiologic arousal, resulting in a complaint of sleeplessness and decreased daytime functioning. For simplification purposes, the term **insomnia** will be used throughout this chapter to refer to psychophysiologic or primary insomnia.

Note that for a diagnosis of insomnia, the individual child or adolescent must make the complaint of insomnia. Thus, for difficulties initiating and/or maintaining sleep in younger children, which typically involves a parental complaint of sleeplessness in the child, see Chapters 6 and 7 regarding bedtime difficulties and nightwakings.

Insomnia

Insomnia involves difficulty falling asleep and/or maintaining sleep, including early morning awakenings. In many cases, insomnia is a symptom secondary to another sleep or medical disorder. In contrast, *primary insomnia* is accompanied by learned sleep-preventing associations and physiological arousal, resulting in a complaint of sleeplessness and decreased daytime functioning.

EPIDEMIOLOGY

- **Prevalence.** No studies have been conducted on the prevalence of insomnia in normal populations of either school-aged children or adolescents. However, several studies report a prevalence of 12% to 33% of adolescents who state that they are "poor sleepers."
- **Gender.** Studies with adults note that the complaint of insomnia is more common in women than men.

ETIOLOGY/RISK FACTORS

There are a number of theories as to the mechanism of primary insomnia. Factors that have been studied include physiologic arousal, emotional arousal, cognitive arousal, and faulty conditioning; however, empirical evidence is inconclusive. The two factors that are the most substantiated are:

- **Sleep behaviors** (maladaptive sleep habits), including excessive time in bed, irregular sleep–wake schedules, and daytime napping.
- **Sleep cognitions** (beliefs and attitudes about sleep), such as "I'll never be able to fall asleep tonight."

Insomnia most likely results from a combination of *predisposing* factors (such as genetic vulnerability, underlying medical or psychiatric conditions) with *precipitating* factors (acute stress) and *perpetuating* factors (poor sleep habits, caffeine use, maladaptive cognitions about sleep).

In adults, a number of predisposing risk factors for insomnia have been identified:

- **Personality traits:**
  - **Hyperarousal** (e.g., racing thoughts, increased vigilance)
  - **Obsessional thinking style** ("I can never fall asleep easily")
  - **Repression of emotions**
- **Medical/psychological problems** (e.g., congestive heart failure, chronic obstructive pulmonary disease, anxiety disorders, depression).
- **Gender.** Women are more at risk for developing insomnia.
- **Family history.** It is more likely that the insomnia is based on learned maladaptive sleep habits, but there may be a genetic contribution in some cases.

PRESENTATION

- **Sleep complaints.** The insomnia may present as difficulty falling asleep, difficulty maintaining sleep, or early morning awakenings. Thus, overall sleep efficiency (time asleep divided by time in bed) is reduced.
- **Learned sleep-preventing associations.** Insomnia, by definition, involves learned sleep-preventing associations. These may present as:
  - Excessive daytime worrying about being unable to fall asleep or stay asleep.
  - Trying too hard to fall asleep at bedtime, although sleep comes easily at other times (e.g., while watching television).
  - Increased somatic tension related to sleep, including agitation or muscle tension.

- **Decreased daytime functioning.** Insomniacs often complain of subjective cognitive impairment and poor functioning.

Associated Features

- **Changes in mood** and decreased sense of well-being.
- **Daytime fatigue,** although rarely excessive daytime sleepiness.
- **Poor school performance**, related to decreased mood and fatigue.
- **Excessive caffeine use,** to maintain wakefulness and combat daytime fatigue.
- **Hypnotic use,** including prescription or over-the-counter hypnotics (e.g., antihistamine preparation), is common in adults with insomnia and may be present in adolescent and college-aged patients.

Diagnostic Criteria

See Tables 17.1 and 17.2.

TABLE 17.1. *Diagnostic criteria (ICSD): psychophysiologic insomnia (307.42)*

A. A complaint of insomnia is present and is combined with a complaint of decreased functioning during wakefulness.
B. Indications of learned sleep-preventing associations are found and include the following:
   1. Trying too hard to sleep, suggested by an inability to fall asleep when desired, but ease of falling asleep during other relatively monotonous pursuits, such as watching television or reading.
   2. Conditioned arousal to bedroom or sleep-related activities, indicated by sleeping poorly at home but sleeping better away from home or when not carrying out bedtime routines.
C. There is evidence that the patient has increased somatized tensions (e.g., agitation, muscle tension, or increased vasoconstriction).
D. Polysomnographic monitoring demonstrates all of the following:
   1. An increased sleep latency
   2. Reduced sleep efficiency
   3. An increased number and duration of awakenings
E. No other medical or mental disorder accounts for the sleep disturbance.
F. Other sleep disorders can coexist with the insomnia, e.g., inadequate sleep hygiene, obstructive sleep apnea syndrome.

Minimal Criteria: A plus B.
Used with permission from American Academy of Sleep Medicine. *The international classification of sleep disorders, revised: diagnostic and coding manual.* Westchester, IL: AASM, 1997: 31–32.

TABLE 17.2. *Diagnostic criteria (DSM-IV): primary insomnia*

A. The predominant complaint is difficulty initiating or maintaining sleep, or nonrestorative sleep, for at least 1 month.
B. The sleep disturbance (or associated daytime fatigue) causes clinically significant distress or impairment in social, occupational, or other important areas of functioning.
C. The sleep disturbance does not occur exclusively during the course of narcolepsy, breathing-related sleep disorder, circadian rhythm sleep disorder, or a parasomnia.
D. The disturbance does not occur exclusively during the course of another mental disorder (e.g., major depressive disorder, generalized anxiety disorder, delirium).
E. The disturbance is not due to the direct physiological effects of a substance (e.g., a drug of abuse, a medication) or a general medical condition.

American Psychiatric Association. *Diagnostic and statistical manual of mental disorders, fourth edition (DSM-IV).* Washinton, DC: American Psychiatric Press, 1994:557.

EVALUATION

- **Medical history:** A thorough medical history should include evaluation of other possible causes of sleep onset difficulties, such as symptoms of obstructive sleep apnea, restless legs syndrome, psychiatric disorders, and alcohol and drug use. Chronic and acute medical conditions may exacerbate primary insomnia symptoms. Concurrent medications should be reviewed as possible contributory factors, especially psychostimulants. Caffeine use and cigarette smoking may also play a role.
- **Developmental/school history:** Generally normal. Adolescents with primary insomnia tend to have anxious or obsessional personality traits and are often academic "overachievers." This situation may lead to a cycle of heightened anxiety about the effects of the insomnia on academic performance and even more difficulty falling asleep.
- **Family history:** Symptoms are often present in first-degree relatives, which may be an indication of genetic vulnerability and/or environmental modeling.
- **Behavioral assessment:** May reveal mood disturbances and anxiety disorders.
- **Physical examination:** Usually unremarkable.
- **Diagnostic tests:**
  - **Sleep diaries** will reveal prolonged sleep onset and/or nighttime awakenings and/or early morning awakenings. Sleep diaries often yield important additional information on maladaptive bedtime activities and behaviors when insomnia is suspected. Sometimes, sleep diaries may indicate that the patient's *subjective* perception of sleep difficulty is actually significantly worse than the sleep log evidence would suggest (termed *sleep state misperception*).
  - **Polysomnography** is rarely indicated in the evaluation of insomnia unless an additional underlying sleep disorder is suspected.

DIFFERENTIAL DIAGNOSIS

Insomnia, as discussed above, is a symptom that can be the result of a number of sleep disorders. Thus, differential diagnosis is critical in the diagnosis of primary insomnia:

- **Transient insomnia.** Transient, or short-term, insomnia typically occurs in individuals with previously normal sleep. Transient insomnia can be the result of sleeping in an unfamiliar or nonconducive (e.g., too noisy, too hot) sleep environment; stressful life event; disruption of sleep schedule (e.g., trip, jet lag); or an illness.
- **Restless legs syndrome/periodic limb movement disorder.** Individuals with restless legs syndrome (see Chapter 14) often present with difficulty falling asleep at bedtime, whereas middle-of-the-night wakings can be associated with periodic limb movement disorder. The key differentiation between insomnia and these disorders is the reporting of uncomfortable sensations in the legs when trying to fall asleep with restless legs syndrome and restlessness/leg movements with periodic limb movement disorder.

- **Obstructive sleep apnea.** Sleep disordered breathing may result in difficulties falling asleep and maintaining sleep given the frequent arousals that result from the apneic pauses. Children and adolescents with sleep disordered breathing will likely have additional symptoms, such as snoring, noisy breathing, breathing pauses, and restlessness (see Chapter 13).
- **Delayed sleep phase syndrome.** Delayed sleep phase syndrome results in few or no difficulties falling asleep at the individual's preferred (later) bedtime, whereas patients with insomnia complain of delayed sleep onset no matter what time they go to bed. In addition, when allowed to choose their own schedule, patients with delayed sleep phase syndrome, fall asleep and wake at consistent times. (see Chapter 16).
- **Inadequate sleep hygiene.** Poor sleep habits (see Chapter 18), including maintaining an erratic sleep schedule, or the use of caffeine or other substances, and inadequate sleep can coexist with insomnia, although patients with psychological insomnia often continue to experience sleep disturbances even after maintaining adequate sleep hygiene.
- **Lifestyle issues.** Practices such as staying up late to socialize or engage in other activities (e.g., television viewing) are voluntary behaviors that may result in a an individual's habitually going to bed late.
- **Psychiatric disorders** (e.g., depression, anxiety). In these cases, the sleep disturbance is likely to covary with the symptoms of the psychiatric disorder. Other related psychiatric symptoms, such as vegetative signs (e.g., loss of appetite), are also present. In generalized anxiety disorder, anxiety symptoms are reported both at bedtime and throughout the day, and daytime functioning is impaired. In addition, the anxiety in insomnia is specifically related to the inability to sleep, whereas that associated with generalized anxiety disorder is more global and diffuse. It should be noted that in adults with primary insomnia, a concomitant psychiatric disorder is found in 25% to 30% of cases.
- **Medical factors.** Difficulty falling asleep may be attributed to a primary medical disorder, including asthma, allergies, and headaches (see Chapter 21 for a review of sleep and medical disorders), as well as to associated conditions, such as pain, physical discomfort, or medications.

MANAGEMENT

When to Refer

Children or adolescents with insomnia who also present with symptoms of other underlying sleep disrupters (e.g., obstructive sleep apnea) should be referred to a sleep specialist. Children whose insomnia fails to respond to simple behavioral interventions may also benefit from referral to a sleep clinic or behavioral medicine specialist with expertise in treating sleep problems. If there are concerns regarding psychiatric or psychological issues, a referral to a mental health specialist is warranted.

Treatment

A thorough evaluation for possible causes of and contributing factors to the insomnia is critical prior to the development of a treatment plan. The following treatment strategies can be effective with primary insomnia; however, these strategies can also be beneficial in some cases of secondary insomnia.

- **Sleep hygiene.** Maintenance of appropriate sleep hygiene (see Chapter 18 and patient handouts in Appendices F15 and F16) is critical with insomnia, including:
  - Appropriate and consistent sleep schedule
  - Avoidance of caffeine
  - Sleep-conducive environment
  - Bedtime routine
  - Consistent morning wake time, regardless of the prior night's sleep, to regulate the internal clock and synchronize the sleep–wake cycle
- **Behavioral treatment.** The goal of behavioral interventions is to disrupt the negative learned associations that are often a prominent feature of primary insomnia. These include:
  - **Cognitive restructuring.** This cognitive-behavioral technique involves teaching the patient to counter inappropriate thoughts, using a three-step process: (a) identifying the inappropriate sleep cognition, (b) challenging the validity of each sleep cognition, and (c) replacing the thought with a more productive one.
  - **Relaxation:** Relaxation strategies, primarily progressive muscle relaxation, as well as deep breathing, visual imagery, and meditation can be beneficial.
  - **Sleep restriction.** Restriction of the time in bed to a minimum of hours, usually 6 to 7, will increase sleep efficiency, consolidate sleep, and disrupt the learned association of sleeplessness and being in bed. Consistent and accurate recording of sleep patterns in a sleep diary is an essential component of sleep restriction therapy. To begin, the amount of time in bed should be set to the estimated amount of nighttime sleep at baseline. Once the sleep efficiency (total sleep time/time in bed) is greater than 85%, a schedule of increasing time in bed (which is gradual enough to maintain the sleep efficiency above 85%). is instituted over a period of days to weeks. However, given the potential for daytime impairment, sleep should never be restricted to less than 6 hours in children and adolescents.
  - **Stimulus control.** Stimulus control involves discontinuing any activities in bed that are not conducive to sleep (including watching television, reading, and worrying), as these activities often serve as cues for wakefulness rather than sleepiness. The patient should delay bedtime until he or she is sleepy (e.g., yawning, eyes drooping). Once in bed, the patient should get out of the bedroom if not asleep within 15 to 20 minutes, and engage in a quiet *non-stimulating* activity (e.g., reading). When again drowsy, the patient should return to bed. It may be necessary to repeat this cycle several times. It is crit-

ical for the patient to leave the bedroom if unable to fall asleep or else the cycle will continue, with the bedroom and bed associated with sleeplessness.

• **Medication.** Hypnotics are typically not recommended for insomnia, especially in children and adolescents, other than for occasional use. The hypnotic should only be used on a scheduled basis (e.g., before a final examination) or for one to three nights in an attempt to break the cycle of insomnia. Note that no hypnotics have been studied for use in children and adolescents (see Chapter 19).

PROGNOSIS

Research has not been conducted on the long-term outcome of insomnia in children or adolescents. However, given the persistence of some underlying predisposing factors for insomnia such as certain personality traits, some individuals are clearly at risk for recurrent problems. In addition, the learned nature of the disorder makes it likely that insomnia will persist if untreated.

Tips for Talking to Parents

• **Distinguish between insomnia as a symptom and insomnia as a disorder.**
• **Explain the learned nature of insomnia.**
• **Develop appropriate sleep hygiene.**
• **Discuss treatment options.**

See Appendix F14 for parent handout on insomnia.

18

Insufficient Sleep and Inadequate Sleep Hygiene

Insufficient sleep and **inadequate sleep hygiene** are the most common causes of excessive daytime sleepiness and sleep difficulties.

Insufficient sleep is defined as inadequate nighttime sleep relative to sleep need. The resulting chronic sleep deprivation impacts on daytime functioning and causes excessive daytime sleepiness, which can be manifested in a number of ways in children and adolescents (e.g., falling asleep unintentionally, overactivity, behavior problems).

Insufficient Sleep

Insufficient sleep is the most common cause of excessive daytime sleepiness. The resulting chronic sleep deprivation impacts on daytime functioning, resulting in mood disturbances, daytime behavior problems, cognitive impairment, and increased risk-taking behavior.

Inadequate sleep hygiene includes two categories of sleep-related behaviors: practices that increase arousal and practices that are inconsistent with sleep organization. *Practices that increase arousal* include caffeine intake, evening television viewing, and rough play at bedtime. Other arousing practices include use of bright light in the bedroom during the night or in the early morning, hearing noise from a sibling who shares a bedroom, or playing video games. *Practices that are inconsistent with sleep organization* include napping late in the day, maintaining a disorganized sleep–wake cycle, and spending excessive time in bed in comparison with time asleep. These behaviors can result in difficulties falling asleep at bedtime, nighttime awakenings, and early morning awakenings. Prolonged inadequate sleep hygiene can produce insomnia (see Chapter 17). Conversely, those with insomnia frequently engage in inadequate sleep hygiene practices.

Inadequate Sleep Hygiene

Inadequate sleep hygiene is the most common cause of difficulties initiating and maintaining sleep. It involves practices that increase arousal and are inconsistent with sleep organization.

EPIDEMIOLOGY

Several studies have suggested a high prevalence of insufficient sleep and/or inadequate sleep hygiene in children or adolescents. In addition, reports indicate that a large percentage of adults do not maintain an appropriate sleep schedule or practice good sleep hygiene.

ETIOLOGY/RISK FACTORS

Insufficient sleep
- **Academic and extracurricular demands** can result in delayed bedtimes.
- **Social activities,** such as late-night socializing (including on the Internet), often delay bedtime in older children and adolescents.
- **Television viewing time** and time playing computer and video games, particularly if there is a television set and/or computer in the child's bedroom, may take priority over bedtime in some families.
- **Part-time employment,** especially if more than 20 hours per week, is associated with inadequate sleep in teenagers.
- **Early school start time** is a major risk factor for inadequate sleep in older children and adolescents. Given the need for 9 to 10 hours of sleep in adolescents, coupled with a delayed shift in circadian rhythm, early school start times do not enable most adolescents to obtain adequate sleep on a nightly basis.

Inadequate sleep hygiene
- **Knowledge gaps** (in both children and parents) regarding appropriate (and inappropriate) sleep habits and the consequences of poor sleep.
- **Lack of adequate adult role models** regarding healthy sleep habits.
- **Inadequate parental supervision** of sleep and bedtime behaviors.

PRESENTATION

Insufficient sleep
- **Excessive sleepiness,** including falling asleep at inappropriate times (e.g., falling asleep in school), unplanned naps, or planned naps past an age when napping is appropriate.
- **Associated features**
  - *Mood disturbance,* including complaints of moodiness, irritability, emotional lability, depression, and anger.
  - *Fatigue and daytime lethargy,* including increased somatic complaints (headaches, muscle aches).

- *Cognitive impairment,* including problems with memory, attention, concentration, decision making, and problem solving.
- *Daytime behavior problems,* including overactivity, impulsivity, and noncompliance.
- *Risk-taking behaviors,* especially in adolescents.
- *Academic problems,* including chronic tardiness related to insufficient sleep and school failure resulting from chronic daytime sleepiness.
- *Use of stimulant medications* and other alertness enhancers such as caffeine and nicotine to artificially maintain wakefulness and combat daytime fatigue.

Inadequate sleep hygiene
- **Sleep problems,** including delayed sleep onset, nighttime awakenings, and early morning awakening
- **Associated features**
  - *Mood changes* and decreased sense of well-being.
  - *Excessive daytime sleepiness* including drowsiness and unplanned napping.
  - *Fatigue* and somatic complaints.
  - *Cognitive impairment and poor school performance* related to excessive sleepiness, negative mood, and fatigue.
  - *Caffeine use* and other artificial alertness enhancers to maintain wakefulness and combat daytime fatigue.

Diagnostic Criteria

See Tables 18.1 and 18.2.

TABLE 18.1. *Diagnostic criteria: insufficient sleep (307.49)*

A. The patient has a complaint of excessive sleepiness or, in prepubertal children, of difficulty initiating sleep.
B. The patient's habitual sleep episode is shorter in duration than is expected for his or her age.
C. When the habitual sleep schedule is not maintained (e.g., weekends or vacation time), patients will have a sleep episode that is greater in duration than the habitual sleep episode and will awaken spontaneously.
D. The abnormal sleep pattern is present for at least 3 months.
E. A therapeutic trial of a longer sleep episode eliminates the symptoms.
F. Polysomnographic monitoring performed over the patient's habitual sleep period demonstrates:
  1. Sleep latency less than 15 min, a sleep efficiency greater than 85%, and a final awakening of less than 10 min
  2. An MSLT demonstrates excessive sleepiness
G. No other medical or mental disorders accounts for the sleep disturbance.
H. The patient's symptoms do not meet the criteria for any other sleep disorder producing either insomnia or excessive sleepiness.

Minimal criteria: A plus B plus C plus G plus H.
MSLT, multiple sleep latency test.
Used with permission from American Academy of Sleep Medicine. *The international classification of sleep disorders, revised: diagnostic and coding manual.* Westchester, IL: AASM, 1997: 89–90.

TABLE 18.2. *Diagnostic criteria: inadequate sleep hygiene (307.41)*

A. The patient has a complaint of either insomnia or excessive sleepiness.
B. At least one of the following is present:
1. Daytime napping at least two times each week
2. Variable wake-up times or bedtimes
3. Frequent periods (two to three times per week) of extended amounts of time in bed
4. Routine use of products containing alcohol, tobacco, or caffeine in the period preceding bedtime
5. Scheduling exercise too close to bedtime
6. Engaging in exciting or emotionally upsetting activities too close to bedtime
7. Frequent use of the bed for nonsleep activities (e.g., television watching, reading, studying, snacking)
8. Sleeping on an uncomfortable bed (poor mattress, inadequate blankets, etc.)
9. Allowing the bedroom to be too bright, too stuffy, too cluttered, too hot, too cold, or in some way not conducive to sleep
10. Performing activities demanding high levels of concentration shortly before bed
11. Allowing mental activities such as thinking, planning, reminiscing, to occur in bed
C. Polysomnography demonstrates one or more of the following:
1. Increased sleep latency
2. Reduced sleep efficiency
3. Frequent arousals
4. Early-morning awakening
5. Excessive sleepiness on a multiple sleep latency test
D. No evidence of a medical or mental disorder accounts for the sleep disturbance.
E. No other sleep disorder either produces difficulty in initiating or maintaining sleep or causes excessive sleepiness.

Minimal criteria: A plus B.
Used with permission from American Academy of Sleep Medicine. *The international classification of sleep disorders, revised: diagnostic and coding manual.* Westchester, IL: AASM, 1997: 76–77.

EVALUATION

- **Medical history:** A thorough medical history should include evaluation for other possible causes of daytime sleepiness (e.g., sleep disorders such as sleep disordered breathing, periodic limb movement disorder, and narcolepsy; psychiatric disorders; alcohol and drug use) and sleep onset difficulties (e.g., insomnia, restless legs syndrome). Concurrent medications should be reviewed as possible contributory factors, especially psychostimulants.
- **Developmental/school history:** Generally normal, although academic problems are often present when sleep is generally insufficient to meet sleep needs.
- **Family history:** Other family members often have a history of poor sleep habits and insufficient sleep.
- **Physical examination:** Usually benign.
- **Diagnostic tests:**
  - **Sleep diaries.** Sleep diary data will reveal reduced nighttime sleep, reduced sleep latency, and possible weekend oversleep following insufficient sleep. Prolonged sleep onset and/or nighttime awakenings are indicative of inadequate sleep hygiene.

DIFFERENTIAL DIAGNOSIS

- **Insomnia.** Symptoms of insomnia will typically persist following institution of appropriate sleep hygiene.
- **Restless legs syndrome/periodic limb movement disorder.** Symptoms of restless legs syndrome (see Chapter 14) often present as difficulty falling asleep, whereas middle-of-the-night awakenings can be associated with periodic limb movement disorder. The key differentiation is the reporting of uncomfortable sensations in the legs when trying to fall asleep with restless legs syndrome and restlessness/leg movements with periodic limb movement disorder.
- **Obstructive sleep apnea.** Sleep disordered breathing may result in difficulties falling asleep and maintaining sleep given the frequent arousals that result from the apneic pauses. Parents of children and adolescents with sleep disordered breathing are also likely to report snoring, noisy breathing, breathing pauses, and restlessness (see Chapter 13).
- **Narcolepsy.** Narcolepsy is characterized by uncontrollable bouts of profound sleepiness and short refreshing naps. Other associated symptoms include fragmented nighttime sleep, cataplexy, hypnagogic hallucinations, and sleep paralysis (see Chapter 15).
- **Delayed sleep phase syndrome.** Delayed sleep phase syndrome involves an intractable shift in the circadian clock resulting in a consistent preferred (late) sleep onset and waketime that is highly resistant to change (see Chapter 16).
- **Sleep onset association disorder/limit-setting sleep disorder.** The inability to fall asleep or stay asleep, especially in a younger child, may be the result of negative sleep associations or poor limit setting by parents (see Chapters 6 and 7).
- **Psychiatric disorders** (e.g., depression, bipolar disorder, generalized anxiety disorder). In these cases, the sleep disturbance and daytime sleepiness will likely covary with the symptoms of the psychiatric disorder (see Chapters 17 and 22).
- **Medical factors.** Difficulty falling asleep may be attributed to a primary medical disorder and associated conditions such as pain, physical discomfort, or use of medications (see Chapter 21 for a review of sleep and medical disorders).

MANAGEMENT

When to Refer

Children or adolescents who also present with symptoms of other underlying sleep disrupters (e.g., obstructive sleep apnea) should be referred to a sleep specialist. Where there are concerns regarding psychiatric or psychological issues, a referral to a mental health specialist is warranted.

Treatment

A careful assessment of both the causes of and contributing factors to the sleep difficulties and/or daytime sleepiness is critical prior to the development of a treatment plan.

- **Appropriate sleep schedule.** A sleep schedule that factors in both individual sleep needs and lifestyle issues should be developed with the child or adolescent and the parents.
- **Sleep hygiene** (see patient handouts in Appendices F15 and F16)
  - Appropriate and consistent sleep schedule
  - Avoidance of caffeine
  - Sleep-conducive environment
  - Bedtime routine
  - Consistent morning waketime regardless of the prior night's sleep so as to regulate the internal clock and synchronize the sleep–wake cycle

PROGNOSIS

The prognosis is good with institution of appropriate sleep schedule and positive sleep hygiene.

Tips for Talking to Parents

- **Stress the importance of sleep.**
- **Discuss the consequences of sleep deprivation.**
- **Develop an appropriate sleep schedule,** enlisting the child/adolescent in setting bedtimes and waketimes for both weekdays and weekends.
- **Outline appropriate sleep hygiene.**

See appendix F15 for parent handout on sleep tips for children and F16 on sleep tips for adolescents.

19

Sleep and Medications

MEDICATIONS FOR SLEEP

Although many sleep disturbances in children are appropriately managed with behavioral therapy alone, there may be clinical situations in which pharmacologic intervention or a combination of behavioral and pharmacologic intervention is considered by the pediatric practitioner for *significant difficulties in initiating and maintaining sleep* (medication use for specific sleep disorders such as restless legs syndrome and narcolepsy are covered in their respective chapters). A variety of over-the-counter and prescription medications in the category of *sedatives/hypnotics* are currently in use in clinical practice to treat pediatric "insomnia." It should be reemphasized in the context of the following discussion of medication use that insomnia is a *descriptive* rather than a diagnostic term and does not specify etiology, as there are many possible causes for the same constellation of symptoms (i.e., bedtime resistance and nightwakings).

A host of variables may potentially impact on the *likelihood of medication use* in a given clinical situation. These include:

- **Patient variables,** such as age, presence of comorbid psychiatric/developmental conditions such as attention deficit-hyperactivity disorder (ADHD) and autism/pervasive developmental disorder, blindness or severe visual impairment, presence of chronic medical conditions characterized by chronic pain, or acute medical conditions which require hospitalization.
- **Provider/practice setting variables,** including provider familiarity with behavioral treatment strategies, time, and reimbursement issues.
- **Cultural/societal variables,** such as acceptance of psychotropic use in children in general and acceptance of alternative therapies.

Alternatively, there are a number of reasons why practitioners might be *reluctant to prescribe or recommend medications* for sleep problems in children:

- **Concerns about efficacy,** including development of tolerance to drugs and rebound insomnia once the medication is discontinued.

- **Concerns about safety,** including dependency issues, short- and long-term side effects, effects on sleep architecture, and risk of accidental overdose.
- **Ethical considerations,** such as medicating a "parent problem" and giving the "wrong message" to families about management of sleep issues.

Unfortunately, concerns regarding safety and efficacy are somewhat justified, as pediatric sleep disturbances remain one of the most poorly researched areas in pediatric psychopharmacology. Most of the information available regarding use of these medications is taken from adult data. There have been only a handful of studies that have examined the effectiveness of hypnotic/sedative use in children and adolescents using methodologically sound techniques, and most of these are case reports or small case series. Despite this, a number of studies both in Europe and the United States suggest that prescribing or recommending sedatives/hypnotics for sleep complaints is a relatively common practice among pediatricians and general practitioners, as well as child psychiatrists. They also suggest that even in infants and preschoolers, sleep complaints often dominate the presenting symptoms for which psychotropic medications are prescribed.

Sleeping Pills for Sleepless Nights

Despite the lack of supporting empirical data regarding efficacy, tolerability, and safety of both prescription and nonprescription sedatives/hypnotics in children and adolescents, studies suggest that these types of medications are frequently prescribed or recommended by primary care practitioners.

The few psychopharmacologic studies that have been done on children have examined nonprescription medications for sleep, such as antihistamines (e.g., diphenhydramine) and melatonin, as well as prescription medications such as chloral hydrate, benzodiazepines, phenothiazines (including chlorpromazine, trimeprazine, and niaprazine), and tricyclic antidepressants. Results of these studies, many of which involved a combination of pharmacotherapy and behavioral therapy, are mixed. In one study, medication was more effective than placebo in reducing sleep onset and the number of nightwakings, but not the actual time slept. In another study, clinical improvement was only moderate, with many wakeful nights still occurring. Although treatment response is often more rapid with medication than with behavioral intervention, most studies have failed to demonstrate long-term effects. Alternatively, most studies have not reported significant adverse events.

Faced with what is admittedly inadequate empirical support for the use of sleep medications in children and adolescents coexisting with what is sometimes a pressing clinical need, *how does the pediatric practitioner help fami-*

lies make rational choices regarding medication use? In addition to considering the factors listed above, some additional considerations should be kept in mind:

- **Careful evaluation of the causes of and contributing factors to a sleep disturbance** in the individual child or adolescent is key. First and foremost, selection of specific intervention strategies, including behavioral treatment as well as pharmacologic management, must be *diagnostically driven.* For example, sleep onset delay may be related to limit-setting sleep disorder, restless legs syndrome, or delayed sleep phase syndrome, all of which require very different behavioral and medication management strategies. Diagnostic classification systems, such as the *International Classification of Sleep Disorders* (ICSD), allow sleep disorders in children to be *reliably* described and diagnosed, which then provides a rationale for the use of specific treatment strategies, including pharmacologic ones, in the clinical setting.
- Diagnostic assessment must be combined with a thorough evaluation of the **impact of the sleep disturbance on the child's health and daily functioning.** In particular, possible neurobehavioral signs of daytime sleepiness (e.g., mood changes, attention problems, impulsivity, poor school performance) must be carefully assessed.
- Diagnostic assessment must be combined with a thorough evaluation of the **impact of the sleep disturbance on the family.** Parent/family variables that are important to consider include educational level, parenting skills, household composition, parental stress level and caretaker exhaustion, and previous experience with and acceptability of pharmacologic treatment. There are situations, albeit relatively rare, in which families are so exhausted and overwhelmed by the child's sleep problems that concerns about both safety and parental mental health are warranted. This situation is particularly likely to occur in the setting of other developmental and medical issues.
- **Characteristics of the individual clinical situation** must be reviewed. These include type and severity of the sleep problem, duration, frequency, and previous failed attempts at conventional behavioral therapy.

When to Consider Medications for Sleep

There may be clinical situations in which a combination of the severity, chronicity, and resistance to behavioral treatment of the sleep problem, family variables including stress and parental exhaustion, and characteristics of the child (including comorbid medical and developmental/neurologic issues) may make it appropriate to consider the use of medication, *in combination with behavioral therapy and good sleep hygiene*, for sleep problems in children.

It should be emphasized that, in many cases, the use of medication for sleep problems in children is *initiated by parents* (or by adolescent patients) without the physician's knowledge. Parents may assume that over-the-counter medications, such as Benadryl, commonly utilized to induce sleepiness are harmless. In particular, parents often fail to consider potentially harmful effects of "natural" or herbal preparations such as valerian root and melatonin. Lack of knowledge about possible side effects or about interactions of these over-the-counter medications with other drugs poses a safety threat. For example, parents may not be aware that the active ingredient in Tylenol PM (diphenhydramine) is the same as that in Benadryl. Because parents may be embarrassed about the home use of sedative medications, they may be reluctant to share that information with their health care provider. In addition, adolescent patients may fail to consider use of over-the-counter sleep-aids as "taking any medication" when queried. Thus, maintaining an open and nonjudgmental approach is key to optimal communication and allows for the development of more effective and appropriate treatment strategies in cooperation with the family.

Once the decision to include pharmacologic management has been made, additional specific issues to consider include the following:

- **Potential benefits** of pharmacologic intervention must substantially outweigh the risks. Although no drug currently available is "perfect," agents should be selected to maximize the benefit/risk ratio.
- **Pharmacotherapy combined with behavioral therapy** should be used, as this strategy is far more likely to yield long-term success.
- **Adequate sleep hygiene,** including sufficient sleep, a regular sleep schedule, and appropriate bedtime routines, should be part of every management plan (see Chapter 18).
- **Selection of specific pharmacologic agents** should be made according to the type of sleep problem. For example, primary difficulties with initiating sleep require use of a medication that has a rapid onset of action and a very short half-life, whereas sleep maintenance problems may require a somewhat longer acting agent.
- **Selection of medications should also consider specific patient variables,** such as age, presence of comorbid medical and psychiatric conditions, and use of concomitant medications that may interact with sedatives/hypnotics.
- **Treatment goals** should be clearly outlined and measurable (e.g., sleep onset consistently less than 30 minutes, improvement in mood and attentiveness). The immediate goal of treatment should be to *alleviate* or improve rather than eliminate sleep problems.
- **Duration of therapy** should be the shortest possible time interval to achieve results. The duration of therapy should be discussed and clarified with the family before initiating medication.
- **Dosing should be initiated at the lowest level** likely to be effective and titrated up as necessary.

- **Timing of medication** should minimize "morning hangover" or persistent grogginess. In general, this means choosing an agent with the shortest possible half-life.
- **Side effects** should be reviewed with the family, as well as the child or adolescent as appropriate.
- **Monitoring** of efficacy and side effects should take place frequently and systematically.
- **Particularly in adolescents,** both the possibility of interactions with other substances (e.g., alcohol, marijuana) and the potential for abuse of medications should be considered.
- **Abrupt discontinuation of pharmacotherapy** should be avoided, as this is likely to result in rebound symptoms and changes in sleep architecture. In some cases, as with the antihypertensive α agonist clonidine, abrupt discontinuation may be dangerous (rebound hypertension).

SPECIFIC MEDICATIONS COMMONLY USED FOR PEDIATRIC INSOMNIA

It should be kept in mind that most of the information given below is extrapolated from adult data *and there are currently no sleep medications labeled for use in children by the U.S. Food and Drug Administration.* Most manufacturers do not list pediatric soporific doses for these drugs, so that dosing in clinical practice is often based on a relative percentage of the adult dose. Efficacy, tolerability, and safety of these drugs in children are largely unknown. With the exception of the few studies cited above, recommendations for use are based on anecdotal clinical experience. *Currently, there is no ideal hypnotic that has been adequately studied for use in children.*

(Note: Medications are presented in alphabetical order.)

Antihistamines

- **Possible clinical uses:** Reduction of sleep onset latency and nightwakings in normal and neurologically impaired children.
- **Mechanism of action:** Binds to central nervous system (CNS) H₁ subtype histamine receptor.
- **Pharmacokinetics:** First-generation (but not second- and third-generation) agents penetrate the blood–brain barrier at therapeutic doses; rapid absorption.
- **Effects on sleep architecture:** Decreases sleep onset latency; may impair sleep quality.
- **Side effects:** Daytime drowsiness; appetite loss, nausea, vomiting, constipation; cholinergic effects (dry mouth); may cause paradoxical behavioral excitation; overdose may cause hallucinations, convulsions, fixed and dilated pupils.

- **Drug interactions:** Effects potentiated by alcohol, CNS depressants (barbiturates, opiates).
- **Comments:** In general, antihistamines are weak soporifics and anxiolytics; however, parental familiarity with these medications, and thus, acceptance of them tends to be high.

Benzodiazepines

- **Possible clinical uses:** Suppression of partial arousal parasomnias (especially sleep terrors); blind and neurologically impaired children with sleep disturbances; restless legs syndrome; periodic limb movement disorder.
- **Mechanism of action:** Binds to central γ-aminobutyric acid (GABA) receptors.
- **Pharmacokinetics:** Rapid onset of action, usually within 1 hour; food slows absorption; varies in duration of elimination half-lives.
- **Effects on sleep architecture:** suppresses slow-wave sleep and variable REM sleep suppression, reduces frequency of arousals between sleep stages.
- **Side effects:** Daytime drowsiness, cognitive impairment (especially long-acting benzodiazepines), anterograde amnesia or memory loss during the time period between dose and sleep onset (especially short-acting benzodiazepines); impairment of respiratory function (may worsen obstructive sleep apnea symptoms); suppression of muscle activity may improve restless legs syndrome symptoms; marked abuse potential; discontinuation may result in rebound insomnia (especially short-acting benzodiazepines); withdrawal effects include insomnia exacerbation, nightmares, increased arousals, photophobia, and seizures (dose dependent).
- **Drug interactions:** May potentiate effects of alcohol and barbiturates.
- **Comments:** May mask rather than improve sleep symptoms; may induce tolerance; may result in rebound increase in partial arousal parasomnias after discontinuation.

Chloral Hydrate

- **Possible clinical uses:** Severe sleep onset delay, especially in neurologically impaired, blind, and developmentally delayed children.
- **Mechanism of action:** Unknown; interaction with GABA receptors?
- **Pharmacokinetics:** Onset of action within 30 minutes; converted in liver to active metabolite, trichloroethanol; peak concentration and half-life decreases with increasing age (half-life in infants three to four times higher than in adults); longer half-life may be associated with prolonged side effects.
- **Effects on sleep architecture:** Decreases sleep onset latency.
- **Side effects:** Gastrointestinal distress, nausea, vomiting (especially when taken on empty stomach), liver toxicity; dizziness, light-headedness; respiratory depression reported; rarely disorientation, confusion, paranoia; discontinuation after prolonged use may precipitate withdrawal (delirium and seizures); overdose associated with CNS depression and cardiac arrhythmias.

- **Drug interactions:** Other drugs with respiratory depressant effects; CNS depression increases with alcohol, benzodiazepines, and barbiturates.
- **Formulations/dosage:** Capsules, syrup, suppository; usual dose 50 to 75 mg/kg up to maximum of 1 to 2 g per single dose.
- **Comments:** One of the first medications used as a sedative in children; may be habit-forming and associated with development of tolerance; can trigger partial arousal parasomnias, including sleepwalking and sleep terrors.

Clonidine

- **Possible clinical uses:** Sleep onset delay, especially in ADHD; neurologically impaired children.
- **Mechanism of action:** Central α_2-adrenergic receptor agonist; decreases norepinephrine release.
- **Pharmacokinetics:** Rapid absorption, high bioavailability; onset of action within 1 hour, peak effects within 2 to 4 hours; half-life 6 to 24 hours; narrow therapeutic index.
- **Effects on sleep architecture:** Reduces sleep onset latency, increases slow-wave sleep, suppresses REM sleep, discontinuation may lead to REM rebound.
- **Side effects:** Dry mouth; bradycardia, hypotension; irritability and dysphoria; reported to increase partial arousal parasomnias and nightmares (discontinuation); tolerance tends to develop, necessitating dose increases; rebound hypertension and dysphoria on abrupt discontinuation; overdose results in bradycardia, CNS depression, hypotension, respiratory depression, and arrhythmias.
- **Drug interactions:** May interact with other CNS depressants; concerns about possible cardiovascular effects in combination with psychostimulants; need for baseline electrocardiogram (ECG) to assess for possible underlying cardiac conduction effects.
- **Formulations/dosage:** Oral, transdermal patch (for daytime symptoms of ADHD, hypertension); reported dosing range for bedtime use 50 to 800 μg (mean 157 μg); treatment generally starts at 25 to 50 μg (one quarter to one half of 0.1-mg tablet) and is increased by 50-μg increments.
- **Comments:** Both use in clinical practice and reports of pediatric overdose have risen dramatically over the past decade; originally developed as a nasal decongestant; used for hypertension in adults; used to treat daytime symptoms of hyperactivity and impulsivity in ADHD; appears to be highly effective in reducing sleep onset delay in children with ADHD by parental report.

Melatonin

- **Possible clinical uses:** Circadian rhythm disturbances related to blindness, autism/pervasive developmental delay, neurologic impairment, or congenital syndromes such as Rett syndrome; possibly normal children for delayed sleep phase syndrome; "jet lag" (in adults).
- **Mechanism of action:** Mimics effects of endogenous pineal hormone in modulating circadian sleep–wake cycles.

- **Pharmacokinetics:** Little information in children: plasma levels peak 1 hour after administration; soporific effects within 1 to 2 hours.
- **Effects on sleep architecture:** Reduces sleep onset latency (some hypnotic effect); major effect on circadian system.
- **Side effects:** Largely unknown; hypotension, bradycardia, reduction core body temperature; nausea, headache, light-headedness; may lower seizure threshold; potential suppression of hypothalamic gonadal axis theoretically may result in induction of precocious puberty upon withdrawal.
- **Drug interactions:** Largely unknown; nonsteroidal anti-inflammatories, alcohol, caffeine, and benzodiazepines may interfere with melatonin production in the body.
- **Formulations/dosages:** Oral tablets; preparations vary in strength, reliability of dosing, and purity; dosing range reported 0.5 to 10 mg in children and up to 25 mg in adults; may start with 1 mg in younger children, 2.5 to 3 mg in older children, and 5 mg in adolescents; jet lag suggested dosage in adults 3 to 5 mg taken for 3 to 5 days one hour before desired bedtime upon arrival.
- **Comments:** Widely available over-the-counter; often used inappropriately for non-circadian-mediated sleep onset problems; despite multiple caveats, may have utility in the short-term treatment of circadian rhythm disturbances in normal children and adolescents and in the longer term treatment of neurologically impaired children and adolescents.

Trazadone (Desyrel)

- **Possible clinical uses:** Sleep onset delay.
- **Mechanism of action:** 5-Hydroxytryptamine (5-HT, serotonin) agonist, affects action of serotonin.
- **Pharmacokinetics:** Short elimination half-life.
- **Effects on sleep architecture:** Reduces sleep onset latency and improves sleep continuity; suppresses REM sleep, and increases slow-wave sleep.
- **Side effects:** Daytime somnolence; risk of priapism in males.
- **Formulations/dosage:** Usual hypnotic adult dose 25 to 50 mg at bedtime.
- **Comments:** One of the most sedating antidepressant drugs.

Zolpidem (Ambien)/Zaleplon (Sonata)

- **Possible clinical uses:** Widely used as short-acting hypnotic in adults; possible use in adolescents with primary insomnia.
- **Mechanism of action:** High-affinity benzodiazepine receptor agonists: binds to GABA receptors.
- **Pharmacokinetics:** Maximum plasma concentration of zolpidem in 30 to 60 minutes; 2.4 hour half-life; no accumulation with repeated dosing; clinical effects generally within one half hour.
- **Effects on sleep architecture:** Does not appear to alter significantly.
- **Side effects:** Minimal residual daytime effects; daytime drowsiness, dizziness, "drugged" feeling, confusion, anterograde amnesia; little rebound insomnia,

development of tolerance, withdrawal reported in adults; headache; drowsiness and rare respiratory depression/coma with overdose.

- **Formulations/dosage:**
  - Zolpidem: oral tablets; adult dose 10 mg 30 minutes before bedtime.
  - Zaleplon: oral tablets; adult dose 5 to 10 mg.
- **Comments:** Appear to be relatively safe, well-tolerated, and effective in adults for short-term use in insomnia; little experience in children or adolescents.

There is currently no "ideal" pediatric sedative/hypnotic that has been adequately tested for use in children.

Herbal preparations may be used to increase wakefulness, as well as to induce sleep. Table 19.1 lists some of the more common preparations, active compounds, and typical uses. Many of the stimulant herbal preparations, including herbal teas, and weight loss and laxative preparations, contain a significant

TABLE 19.1. *Herbal stimulants and sedatives*

Common name	Scientific name and plant family genus, species, author of name (family)	Active compounds	Typical uses
Guarana	*Paullinia* Cupana Kunth (Sapindaceae)	Caffeine	Stimulant
Yerba mate	*Ilex Paraguariensis* St.-Hil (Aquifoliaceae)	Caffeine	Stimulant
Ephedra Ma Huang	*Ephedra sinica* L. (Ephedraceae)	Ephedrine Pseudoephedrine	Stimulant, asthma, nasal congestion, weight loss
Indian Sida	*Sida Cordifolia* L. (Malvacene)	Ephedrine	Stimulant, nasal congestion
Bitter orange	*Citrus Aurantium* L. (Rutacene)	Synephrine	Stimulant, weight loss
Yohimbe	*Pausinystlia Johimbe* Pierre ex Beille (Rubiaceae)	Yohimbine	Stimulant, body building, aphrodisiac
Valerian	*Valeriana Officinalis* L. (Valerianaceae)	Valepotriates? Valerenic acid?	Sedative
German chamomile	*Matricaria recutita* Raeusch. (Asteraceae)	Apigenin	Mild sedative, gastrointestinal complaints, inflammation
Kava	*Piper Methysticum* L. (Piperaceae)	Kavalactones (Kavapyrones)	Anxiolytic, muscle relaxant
Lavender	*Lavandula Angustifolia* Miller (Larniaceae)	Linaloyl acetate, Linalool	Sedative, upper abdominal complaints
Hops	*Humulus Lupulus* L. (Cannabinaceae)	2-methyl-3-buten-2-ol	Mild sedative
Lemon balm	*Melissa Officinalis* L. (Lamiaceae)	Not determined	Mild sedative
Passiflora, passion flower	*Passiflora incarnata* L. (Passifloraceae)	Harman alkaloids? Chrysin?	Mild sedative

percentage of caffeine. **Valerian root,** which has benzodiazepine-like properties, has been shown in several studies in adults to have sleep-promoting effects without the "hangover" effects seen with the benzodiazepines, although effects may not be seen for several weeks. **Chamomile** is reported anecdotally to have mild sedating effects; **kava** has been studied in both anxiety and insomnia with some improvement in subjective sleep parameters and little negative impact on performance. **Lavender** appears to have a CNS depressive effect and as such may potentiate the effects of other CNS depressants such as alcohol; aromatherapy with the volatilized oil has been reported to improve sleep quality.

MEDICATION EFFECTS ON SLEEP

Many over-the-counter and prescription drugs have profound effects on sleep in adults. Although these effects are much less well studied in children and adolescents, certain basic pharmacologic principles may be applied to both adults and children. Drugs may exert their effects on sleep in several ways:

- **Direct** pharmacologic effect
- Disturbance in **sleep patterns** (e.g., nightmares)
- Exacerbation of a **primary sleep disorder** (e.g., obstructive sleep apnea and restless legs syndrome)
- **Drug withdrawal** effects
- **Daytime sleepiness**

Understanding a medication's effects on *sleep architecture* (either direct or in withdrawal) can help predict the likely clinical effect on sleep:

- **Decreased slow-wave sleep (SWS)** may lead to subjective feelings of "not being well-rested".
- **Increased SWS** may increase partial arousal parasomnias in susceptible individuals.
- **Decreased REM sleep** may result in increased parasomnias.
- **Increased REM sleep** may result in increased nightmares.

Drug effects on various *neurotransmitters* of sleep and wakefulness may also be responsible for their clinical effects. For example, GABA agonists like benzodiazepines promote sleep (increase non-REM sleep), whereas adenosine receptor blockers like caffeine promote wakefulness (inhibit non-REM sleep).

Specific Effects of Commonly Used Drugs in Pediatrics on Sleep

Alcohol: Frequently used to promote sleep. However, despite the fact that alcohol decreases sleep onset latency, it may also cause significantly decreased sleep continuity and sleep disruption; *"biphasic"* effect on sleep architecture: increases slow-wave sleep and suppresses REM sleep in the first part of the night, but, as alcohol levels decline, results in REM rebound, decreased slow-wave sleep, and sleep fragmentation; exacerbates partial arousal parasomnias (increases slow-wave sleep) and nightmares (REM rebound) as well as restless legs syndrome symptoms and obstructive sleep apnea symptoms; acute withdrawal associated with increased wakefulness, increased REM sleep, and decreased slow-wave sleep.

Anticonvulsants:
- **Carbamazepine (Tegretol):** Associated with increased daytime somnolence; may decrease sleep onset latency.
- **Phenobarbital:** Tends to be very sedating, dose dependent, with some development of tolerance over time; decreases sleep onset latency
- **Phenytoin (Dilantin):** May cause less daytime sleepiness than other anticonvulsants.
- **Valproic Acid (Depakote):** Associated with increased daytime somnolence; no reported major direct effects on sleep.
- **Newer anticonvulsants:** These medications have varying degrees of daytime sedation; topiramate (Topamax) 15% to 25%, gabapentin (Neurontin) 5% to 15%; tends to improve over time; direct effects on sleep are largely unknown.

Antidepressants: Most antidepressants, especially those with anticholinergic effects, suppress REM and increase latency to REM sleep; abrupt withdrawal may lead to increased nightmares (REM rebound).
- **Bupropion (Wellbutrin):** Insomnia reported in 5% to 19% adults; increases REM sleep and reduces REM onset latency.
- **Selective serotonin reuptake inhibitors, or SSRIs (Prozac, Paxil, Zoloft):** Often activating; frequent reports of sleep disruption in adults; increases sleep onset latency; suppresses REM sleep; may also cause daytime sedation. May worsen RLS symptoms. Newer generation SSRI medications such as **citalopram (Celexa)** appear to have fewer sleep-disrupting effects and may be useful in the management of insomnia associated with depression.
- **Tricyclic antidepressants:** May be used to treat insomnia associated with depression because of decreased sleep onset latency and decreased arousals during sleep stage transitions. Also used to treat partial arousal parasomnias due to direct effects (decrease) on slow-wave sleep. Withdrawal may lead to REM rebound (increased nightmares) and slow-wave sleep rebound (increased partial arousal parasomnias). May exacerbate restless legs syndrome symptoms. Tend to increase daytime somnolence (amitriptyline, doxepin, and trimipramine more sedating; imipramine, desipramine, nortriptyline, amoxapine moderately sedating).
- **Venlafaxine (Effexor):** May cause difficulty initiating and maintaining sleep, as well as result in daytime somnolence.
- **Other newer antidepressants: Nefazadone (Serzone)** and **mirtazapine (Remeron):** Less likely to cause insomnia, particularly in comparison to most of the SSRIs. They may result in daytime somnolence (especially mirtazapine).

Antihistamines: First-generation drugs (diphenhydramine, hydroxyzine, chlorpheniramine) cross blood–brain barrier and promote sleep; sleep onset latency is shortened, but there appears to be few direct effects on sleep architecture. They may also significantly reduce daytime alertness and impair performance (second and third generation, such as terfenadine and loraditine, do not). H_2 receptor blockers (cimetidine) are not widely distributed in the CNS and thus have few sleep effects.

Antipsychotics: "Traditional" drugs [e.g., thioridazine (Mellaril),] associated with increased daytime somnolence; newer agents [risperidone (Risperdal), olanzapine (Zyprexa)] tend to be less sedating, although clozapine (Clozaril) has a high incidence of sedation. Most antipsychotics increase daytime somnolence, decrease sleep onset latency, increase sleep continuity, and suppress REM sleep (higher doses); may promote sleep by attenuating psychiatric symptoms that interfere with sleep.

Barbiturates: Increase daytime somnolence, decrease sleep onset latency; increase sleep continuity, suppress REM sleep and increase REM onset latency; may worsen obstructive sleep apnea symptoms.

β Agonists: May reduce nocturnal arousals.

Corticosteroids: Use associated with insomnia in asthma and cancer patients; subjective increases in wakefulness; decreases REM sleep (hydrocortisone); inhaled steroids do not appear to have significant sleep effects.

Decongestants (pseudoephedrine/phenylpropanolamine): May cause insomnia; may increase plasma caffeine levels.

Lithium: May improve nocturnal sleep, increases daytime sleepiness, increases slow-wave sleep, variable suppression of slow-wave sleep and REM sleep.

Methylxanthines:

- **Theophylline:** Use associated with increased sleep complaints (difficulty falling asleep, disrupted sleep) in those with asthma in comparison with other medications; however, alleviation of nocturnal asthma symptoms may improve sleep quality.

- **Caffeine:** Increases alertness by blocking the sedative effects of the neuromodulator adenosine and increasing excitatory neurotransmitter release. Increased consumption associated with decreased daytime sleepiness/increased alertness; degree of impact on sleep onset latency, sleep disruption, and nonrestorative sleep is dose dependent, although sensitivity to these effects may vary across individuals. Caffeine may exacerbate restless legs syndrome symptoms. Many products contain caffeine (Table 19.2), including a number of over-the-counter cold remedies, pain relievers, and weight loss preparations. There are a number of herbal stimulants (see above) that also contain caffeine as the active ingredient.

Nicotine: Cigarette smoking associated with increased sleep onset latency and disrupted nonrestorative sleep; increases restless legs symptoms, and increases risk of sleep disordered breathing; withdrawal may result in disrupted sleep and daytime somnolence; nicotine gum reduces slow-wave sleep; patch

TABLE 19.2. *Caffeine intake*

Caffeine can result in difficulties initiating and maintaining sleep, and thus a thorough review of substances that contain caffeine is beneficial.

Product	Serving size	Caffeine content (mg)
Coca-cola	8 oz	23
Diet Coke	8 oz	31
Diet Pepsi	8 oz	24
Pepsi	8 oz	25
Dr. Pepper/Diet Dr. Pepper	8 oz	28
Mountain Dew/Diet Mountain Dew	8 oz	37
Sunkist orange soda	8 oz	28
Tab	8 oz	47
Red Bull	330 mL	80
Arizona Blue Luna iced coffees	8 oz	40–50
Cappucino	6 oz	35
Coffee, decaf.	8 oz	5
Starbucks coffee, grande	16 oz	550
Starbucks coffee, short	8 oz	250
Starbucks coffee, tall	12 oz	375
Iced tea	8 oz	25
Mistic teas	8 oz	17
Snapple iced tea (all kinds)	8 oz	21
Baker's chocolate	1 oz	26
Chocolate milk	8 oz	5
Dark chocolate, semisweet	1 oz	20
Coffee ice cream	8 oz	58
Anacin	2 tablets	65
Dexatrim	1 tablet	200
Excedrin, max. strength	2 tablets	130
Midol	1 tablet	32
No Doz, max. strength; Vivarin	1 tablet	200
No Doz, regular strength	1 tablet	100

reduces sleep efficiency (time asleep/time in bed) and prolongs sleep onset latency.

Opioids: Use often results in daytime sedation; disrupts sleep continuity, suppresses REM sleep and slow-wave sleep; may worsen obstructive sleep apnea; suppression of muscle activity may result in improvement in restless legs syndrome symptoms; abrupt discontinuation may lead to insomnia and nightmares.

Stimulants:

- **Amphetamines:** Direct effects include increased wakefulness (use in treating narcolepsy), increased sleep onset latency, decreased total sleep time, suppressed REM sleep, and variable decrease in slow-wave sleep; rebound effect late in the day may result in increased sleep onset latency; discontinuation after prolonged therapy may cause rebound increases in REM sleep, slow-wave sleep, and subjective sleepiness.

Methylphenidate: Direct effects include increased wakefulness (use in treating narcolepsy), decreased total sleep time, decreased sleep continuity, suppression of REM sleep; rebound effect late in the day may result in increased sleep onset latency; in abuse situations, withdrawal may result in severe hypersomnia and REM rebound.

20

Sleep in Special Needs Children

GENERAL CONSIDERATIONS

Sleep disturbances in pediatric special needs populations are extremely common and often a source of considerable stress for the families of these children. The types of sleep disorders that occur in these children are generally not unique to these populations; rather, they are more common and more severe than in the general population. They typically reflect the child's developmental level rather than the chronologic age. Sleep problems, especially in children with special needs, are often chronic in nature and unlikely to resolve without aggressive treatment. Multiple sleep disorders also are likely to occur concurrently. Furthermore, the impact of disrupted and/or inadequate sleep on cognitive, emotional, and social development and behavior in these already at-risk children is potentially profound.

Sleep Screening in Special Needs Children

The high prevalence of sleep disturbances in developmentally delayed children underscores the role of ongoing screening for sleep problems in these populations. In addition, practitioners need to consider multiple factors in evaluating an individual special needs child with a sleep disturbance. The heterogeneity of possible etiologies for and contributing factors to sleep disorders in this population is considerable, and successful treatment is contingent on identifying and addressing these multiple issues.

ETIOLOGY/RISK FACTORS

Some sleep disorders are more commonly associated with specific neurodevelopmental disorders or syndromes, such as obstructive sleep apnea in Down syndrome and circadian rhythm disturbances in blindness. More nonspecific problems, such as shortened sleep duration, irregular sleeping patterns, delayed sleep onset, frequent nightwakings, and early morning waking, are more common across the spectrum of neurodevelopmental disorders. Many children with developmental delays and other special needs have additional risk factors that may predispose them, in general, to sleep disorders. These include:

- **Medical issues**
  - **Craniofacial abnormalities,** such as midface hypoplasia or the micrognathia associated with Pierre Robin syndrome, may predispose a child to sleep disordered breathing.
  - **Obesity,** associated with Prader-Willi and other congenital syndromes, significantly increase the risk of obstructive sleep apnea.
  - **Seizure disorders** may disrupt nocturnal sleep.
  - **Brain malformations** or injuries that affect structures involved in control of sleep–wake rhythms (thalamus, basal forebrain) or respiration (brainstem) increase the likelihood of sleep disturbances.
  - **Muscle disease,** such as congenital myopathies, muscular dystrophies, and hypotonia, increase the likelihood of obstructive sleep apnea and sleep disordered breathing.
  - **Medication use,** including anticonvulsants and psychotropics, may also result in altered sleep patterns and sleep disturbance.
- **Sensory deficits.** Sensory deficits can significantly impact sleep. For example, visual impairment involving complete lack of light perception is associated with profound sleep disturbances, presumably due to alterations in the normal suppression of melatonin by ambient light. Lack of sensitivity to social and environmental cues and heightened/altered sensitivity to sensory stimuli in children with autism and other forms of pervasive developmental disorder may lead to difficulties in settling and problematic nightwakings.

Sleep and the "Out-of-Sync" Child

Although the diagnostic entity known as sensory integration disorder is somewhat controversial, there is no question that children with developmental delays, as well as "normal" children, may experience hypo- or hypersensitivity to environmental stimuli (e.g., sounds, bright lights, labels and seams on clothing, food textures) that may interfere with sleep. Occupational therapy techniques that have been used to address sensory integration issues (e.g., brushing, weighted vests, "white noise" generators, body pillows) may be useful in alleviating sleep onset problems in these children. Evaluation and consultation with a pediatric occupational therapist also may be helpful.

- **Daytime behavioral problems.** Daytime behavior problems, such as aggression and noncompliance, may result in similar behaviors during sleep time, such as bedtime resistance and prolonged nightwakings. In addition, self-injurious behavior has been reported both to result from and to be exacerbated by sleep problems.
- **Cognitive impairment.** Higher degrees of cognitive impairment tend to be associated with more frequent and severe sleep problems, although sleep problems in autism have also been reported to be unrelated to or even associated with a *higher* IQ. Children who have difficulty communicating their needs or understanding and responding to environmental demands are more likely to have problematic sleep. In addition, children with social interaction impairments may be more prone to behavioral sleep disorders
- **Comorbid psychiatric disorders.** Psychiatric disorders such as depression and anxiety are common in children and adolescents with developmental delays and autistic spectrum disorders, and may contribute to sleep problems. Severe hyperactivity/attention deficit-hyperactivity disorder and/or mood instability is common to many chromosomal and genetic disorders, including velocardiofacial syndrome, Angelman syndrome, Williams syndrome, fragile X syndrome, and Klinefelter syndrome, and may contribute to the genesis of sleep onset and maintenance difficulties in these children.
- **Parenting-related variables.** Parenting issues such as difficulty with limit setting and high levels of family stress may contribute to and be exacerbated by sleep difficulties in the developmentally delayed child. Parents of developmentally delayed children may have inappropriate expectations regarding sleep patterns and behaviors that are based on the child's chronologic rather than developmental age. Alternatively, parents may view sleep problems in these children as "inevitable" and, thus, may not actively seek assistance in treating them.
- **Age.** Younger developmentally delayed children are more likely to have sleep issues than older ones.

SPECIFIC DEVELOPMENTAL DELAYS

Specific neurodevelopmental syndromes that have been reported in association with sleep disturbances, including sleep disordered breathing, are listed below.

- **Autism and autism spectrum disorders.** Children with autism and autistic spectrum disorders, such as Asperger syndrome, are prone to a variety of sleep problems, even when compared with children with similar intellectual functioning who are not autistic. These problems are especially likely to occur in children younger than 8 years and include irregular sleep–wake patterns, delayed sleep onset, prolonged nightwakings, short sleep duration, and early and irregular morning waketimes. Nightwakings in these children tend to be longer in duration and more disruptive in terms of behavior. Sleep routines may be more unusual and more problematic in these children because of stereotypic behaviors and difficulties in adapting to any alterations in these routines. In addition to the presence of other risk factors outlined above, some authors have postulated that there may be a primary disturbance of melatonin production and synchronization in autistic children, and some autistic children seem to respond to treatment with exogenous melatonin. Others have suggested that a primary arousal dysfunction in these children contributes to sleep problems. Increased anxiety in these children may also play a role. Finally, some authors who have failed to document objective sleep abnormalities have suggested that parents of autistic children may be more sensitive to and aware of sleep problems in these children.

Sleep in Autism and Pervasive Developmental Disorder

Sleep problems in children with autism and autism spectrum disorders are particularly common. Parents of these children may view the sleep disturbance as "intrinsic" to the disorder and thus may not spontaneously seek medical advice until the problem becomes severe. Sleep problems in these children are often chronic but may be successfully treated with a combination of behavioral and pharmacologic strategies.

- **Williams syndrome.** Williams syndrome is associated with increased periodic limb movement disorder (see Chapter 14).
- **Meningomyelocele and Chiari malformation.** Meningomyelocele (especially thoracic and thoracolumbar) and Chiari malformation type 2 can be associated with blunted ventilatory and arousal responses, central hypoventilation syndrome, and increased central and obstructive apneas.
- **Achondroplasia.** Obstructive sleep apnea (see Chapter 13) is associated with midface hypoplasia and hypotonia.
- **Down syndrome.** Obstructive sleep apnea can be related to hypotonia, central distribution of adipose tissue, glossoptosis, and hypothyroidism. Prevalence of obstructive sleep apnea is reported to be as high as 40%, and does not appear to be related to age or the presence of congenital heart disease. Central apneas are also increased in Down syndrome. Down patients also appear to have more difficulties in initiating sleep, more fragmented sleep in general, and are more likely to have periodic limb movements.
- **Prader-Willi syndrome.** Ventilatory abnormalities (hypoventilation, obstructive sleep apnea, and upper airway resistance syndrome) are associated with obesity but also appear intrinsic to this disorder. Daytime hypersomnolence may occur independent of the presence of sleep disordered breathing.

- **Rett syndrome.** Although ventilatory (hyperventilation and apnea) abnormalities are common during the day, sleep apnea and other sleep-related respiratory disturbances appear to be uncommon in this population. However, these children are more prone to difficulties falling asleep, fragmented sleep, night-wakings, nocturnal events such as night laughing and inconsolable screaming, early morning awakening, and shortened sleep duration.
- **Smith-Magenis syndrome.** In addition to the severe hyperactivity and frequent aggression associated with this syndrome, behavioral sleep problems occur in about 70%.
- **Other developmental delays.** Sleep disordered breathing has also been reported in association with fragile X syndrome and the mucopolysaccharidoses.

Sleep and Breathing in Special Needs Children

Sleep disordered breathing is particularly common in many special needs populations, especially in children who have conditions characterized by midface hypoplasia, hypotonia, and /or obesity. The resulting sleep fragmentation may contribute significantly to learning and behavior problems already present as part of their underlying disorder. Many of these children, once identified, can be successfully treated with continuous positive airway pressure if appropriate behavioral support is available.

EPIDEMIOLOGY

Significant problems with initiation and maintenance of sleep have been reported in a host of different neurodevelopmental disorders, including autism and pervasive developmental delay, Asperger syndrome, Angelman syndrome, tuberous sclerosis, San Filippo syndrome, Rett syndrome, and Williams syndrome. Prevalence of sleep problems in children across the age spectrum with severe mental retardation have been estimated to be on the order of 30% to 80%, and 50% in children with less severe cognitive impairment. Similar estimates in autism are in the 50% to 70% range. Other studies have suggested that similar rates of sleep problems occur in blind children, with difficulty falling asleep, nightwakings, and restless sleep being the most common concerns.

TREATMENT

- **Sleep hygiene.** Basic principles of sleep hygiene in children are particularly important to consider in preventing and treating sleep problems in developmentally delayed children (see Appendices F15 and F16 for sleep hygiene handouts). These include a regular and consistent bedtime, a structured bedtime routine that involves specific and predictable steps, and positive reinforcement for appropriate bedtime behavior. Expectations around nighttime behavior must be clearly communicated and consistently enforced. Encouraging the use of appropriate transitional objects may be particularly important in these children. The development of conditioned associations between the child's bed/bedroom and behaviors incompatible with sleep (playing, watching television) should be avoided. It is also particularly important to maintain a regular daytime routine for mealtime, playtime, and other activities with these children to help synchronize sleep–wake rhythms. Finally, unless developmentally appropriate, daytime sleep periods and naps should be restricted to avoid compromising consolidation of nighttime sleep.

Behavioral Management of Sleep Problems

Sleep disturbances in children with developmental delays are frequently amenable to management with a variety of behavioral strategies. These should be tailored to the developmental level of the child and the resources of the family. Choosing reasonable, attainable, and mutually acceptable target goals in terms of bedtime behaviors, nightwakings, and sleep duration is particularly important in assisting families.

• **Behavioral management.** Children with neurodevelopmental disabilities have many of the same sleep problems as normal children, such as sleep onset association disorder and limit-setting sleep disorder. Therefore, a wide range of behavioral management strategies used in normal children for nightwakings and bedtime resistance, such as sleep scheduling and restriction of daytime sleep, graduated extinction procedures, fading of adult intervention at bedtime and during nightwakings, and positive reinforcement (see Chapters 6 and 7) may also be applied effectively in developmentally delayed children. Bedtime fading, which involves temporarily setting the bedtime at the current sleep onset time and then gradually advancing it to the desired bedtime, may be helpful with sleep onset issues. Not only will these types of behavioral interventions result in improvement in sleep problems for the child, but they may also alleviate parental stress, improve parental sleep, and generalize to improvements in parenting skills and management of daytime behaviors.

Some special considerations should be given to the application of behavioral management strategies in these special populations. Ensuring the safety of these children, especially if nightwaking is a problem or if there is a history of self-injurious behavior, needs to be a key consideration in management. In general, parents tend to be more comfortable with more gradual treatment approaches, especially if there are associated medical issues involved. The severity and chronicity of sleep problems in many of these children often necessitate long-term treatment and utilization of a variety of treatment strategies. In addition, it is particularly important to tailor the behavioral intervention not only to the underlying cause(s) of the sleep disturbance but to the needs and special circumstances of the individual child and family. Finally, collaboration with a behavioral therapist in designing and implementing treatment plans may be prudent if there are complex, chronic, or multiple sleep problems, or if initial behavioral strategies have failed.

- **Pharmacologic treatment.** The use of pharmacologic intervention in conjunction with behavioral techniques has also been shown to be effective in some cases. These include diphenhydramine, chloral hydrate, trazadone, clonidine, and benzodiazepines. The rationale is that the decrease in sleep onset delay associated with short-term use of a short-acting hypnotic medication just before bedtime eliminates prolonged bedtime struggles and increases sleep duration. Parents may then be more successful in implementing bedtime behavioral strategies. Practitioners should be aware of potential pitfalls in using hypnotic medications, including unpredictable side effects in this population, development of tolerance necessitating increasingly higher doses, paradoxical effects (agitation instead of sedation), withdrawal effects and rebound sleep onset delay on discontinuation, and morning "hangover." The last is more likely to occur with use of medications with longer half-life; however, medications with shorter half-life may not be effective in the management of nightwakings.

  Given that children with severe developmental delay and/or neurologic impairment, especially those who are visually impaired, are prone to circadian rhythm or sleep–wake cycle disturbances, a therapeutic role for exogenous melatonin in "resetting" the circadian clock has been proposed. A number of studies have documented improvements in sleep onset delay, nightwakings, early morning waking, and total hours of sleep in up to 80% of children with a variety of disorders (cortical blindness, Rett syndrome, autism, tuberous sclerosis, Asperger syndrome) using a small dose (0.5 to 2.5–5 mg) of melatonin approximately 1 hour before bedtime. Some studies have used doses in the 5- to 10-mg range for refractory cases without reported adverse effects. Melatonin's positive effect on sleep may be due to a combination of its sleep phase setting and hypnotic effects. However, melatonin is not effective in all developmental delayed children with sleep problems, and little is known about long-term side effects. Disadvantages of melatonin include lowering of the seizure threshold, and the theoretical possibility of initiation of precocious puberty if withdrawn abruptly due to effects on the hypothalamic-gonadal axis. Given the over-the-counter availability of melatonin, the purity of preparation and inconsistent dosing are also concerns. Finally, parents may use it inappropriately and without adequate supervision. Overall, melatonin, as with all pharmacologic interventions, is likely to work best in combination with a treatment package that includes a variety of behavioral interventions.

Melatonin

Melatonin is the best-studied pharmacologic intervention for developmentally delayed children with sleep problems and should be seriously considered as an adjunct to behavioral interventions in children with persistent alterations in sleep–wake schedule.

- **Light therapy.** In addition to melatonin, primary circadian rhythm disturbances in these children may also be treated with light therapy and chronotherapy. Morning phototherapy with a light box has been used to successfully treat refractory sleep phase delay in severely brain-damaged children. However, appropriate timing of the phototherapy to achieve the desired shift in sleep–wake phase is key and is best done under the supervision of a sleep professional. Chronotherapy, or the successive delay of the sleep–wake cycle over a period of days until the desired bedtime is reached, has also been used effectively to treat severe sleep onset delay in autistic and blind children. However, it should be kept in mind that sleep–wake cycle disturbances in these children are often accompanied by behavioral problems, especially bedtime resistance, and that successful management of the sleep problem requires attention to both (e.g., avoiding reinforcement of inappropriate bedtime behavior).

  It should also be noted that children who are prone to circadian rhythm disturbances may be relatively sensitive to and disrupted by circadian desynchronization (e.g., jet lag, daylight savings shift). Therefore, parents may need to carefully anticipate these situations.

21

Sleep and Medical Disorders

GENERAL CONSIDERATIONS

Children with both acute and chronic medical conditions may suffer from sleep disturbances, both primary sleep disorders and sleep problems that are secondary to the underlying medical issues. Unfortunately, there have been relatively few studies in the pediatric literature that have examined this issue in detail, so much of the information regarding the types of sleep problems that occur in these children comes from studies of adults with chronic medical conditions or from clinical observations. It is likely that a host of factors contribute to the development and exacerbation of sleep problems in medically compromised children, including physical issues such as pain control and medications, psychological factors such as anxiety and family stress, and environmental variables such as hospitalization. In turn, the effects of sleep fragmentation and sleep deprivation in these children are also likely to be particularly significant, given what is known about the psychological/emotional impact of inadequate sleep and the physiologic effects of sleep deprivation on the immune system and the body's ability to respond to stress.

Sleepiness versus Fatigue

A distinction between sleepiness and fatigue may be relevant in assessing the role of sleep in some medical conditions, although this is sometimes more of a semantic difference that may be difficult to elicit in young children. By definition, "sleepinesss" is the persistent propensity to doze off or fall asleep in inappropriate settings. Although sleepiness may be affected by a host of intervening variables, including time of day, motivation, physiologic states such as hunger, and level of stimulation, true daytime sleepiness generally implies the presence of inadequate and/or disrupted sleep. Fatigue, on the other hand, is more likely to refer to a subjective state of low energy and low motivation, which may or may not primarily be a result of poor sleep.

ETIOLOGIES/RISK FACTORS

• **Pain.** Both acute and chronic pain have major physical and psychological effects on sleep, and these are often bidirectional in nature. Pain may cause sleep onset delay, nightwakings, fragmented and restless sleep, and frequent arousals, as well as daytime fatigue. Even adaptive behaviors, such as protection of the injured area by positioning and increased attention to movements during sleep, may further impact on sleep quality. One study reported that approximately half of a group of children with newly diagnosed cancer suffered pain-related sleep disturbances. Alternatively, the sleepiness and fatigue associated with sleep problems may exacerbate pain. The interaction between pain and sleep is also impacted on by a number of psychological variables. Coping skills needed to deal with pain may be compromised by the mood changes, irritability, low frustration tolerance, and poor regulation of emotions caused by sleep deprivation. Learned associations with both sleep and pain tend to be very powerful, and children may become conditioned to associate bedtime and sleep with negative and painful experiences. Finally, implementation of behavioral management strategies may be impacted by decreased motivation and goal-directed behavior and by decrements in attention and behavioral/impulse control in the sleep-deprived child.

Additional factors that are involved in the complex relationship between sleep and pain include stress, hyperarousal, and anxiety. These may be particularly problematic at sleep onset, which requires not only the relaxation of vigilance and attention to the surrounding environment, but separation from the child's security figures. Sleep may also represent a temporary psychological escape from pain; thus, the inability to initiate or maintain sleep may further heighten anxiety and decrease pain tolerance. Parental anxiety may also compromise caretaker efforts to comfort the child, to set appropriate limits around sleep behavior, and to act as coping role models. Some children with chronic medical conditions associated with pain may have comorbid psychiatric disorders, such as anxiety and depression, which may lead to further deterioration of sleep patterns and quality (see Chapter 22). Children with more acute pain conditions related to trauma may also have posttraumatic stress disorder symptoms that may significantly disrupt sleep.

Finally, medications used for pain management may directly disrupt sleep by affecting sleep patterns and architecture. For example, opiates decrease REM sleep and slow-wave sleep and increase sleep fragmentation. Side effects of analgesics, such as gastrointestinal discomfort, may adversely affect sleep. Withdrawal effects of pain medications may result in sleep disturbances; for example, withdrawal of medications with REM suppressant effects such as benzodiazepines may result in REM sleep rebound and increased nightmares. Finally, inadequate pharmacologic control of nocturnal pain may lead to more disrupted sleep, increased daytime fatigue, and a further deterioration in pain management.

- **Family issues.** Families of children who have had life-threatening illnesses or who have chronic medical conditions may develop a "vulnerable child syndrome," in which parents are unwilling to set limits because of concerns about compromising the child's physical condition. Bedtime resistance and "reactive" co-sleeping with parents may result. In addition, parents may be unwilling to enforce good sleep hygiene rules in children with medical problems, such as regular sleep–wake schedules and avoidance of inappropriate daytime napping, further compounding poor sleep.

- **Hospitalization.** Hospitalization is a stressful event for children and their families, and behavioral regression to a previous developmental level (e.g., dependence on parental presence in order to fall asleep) is a common response, particularly in younger children. This may result in an acute adjustment sleep disorder with difficulties initiating and maintaining sleep and/or may exacerbate preexisting sleep problems. For example, one study reported sleep onset delays resulting in a loss of up to one-fourth of normal sleep time in a group of hospitalized 3- to 8-years-olds. Children with more prolonged and/or life-threatening illnesses requiring frequent hospitalizations, such as cancer, may be even more at risk for chronic sleep disturbances.

  In addition to issues related to the underlying medical condition and family and emotional issues, factors in the hospital environment may contribute significantly to the development of sleep problems in children in the inpatient setting. These factors include noise (including sudden and unexpected noises as well as a high level of background noise); frequent nocturnal interruptions for medication and nursing care; bright and/or inappropriately timed lighting, which may affect the normal circadian release of melatonin and thus further compromise regular sleep patterns; and stress associated with an unfamiliar environment and loss of regular routine. It has been shown that relative sleep loss and sleep fragmentation are particularly common in both adult and pediatric intensive care unit (ICU) settings. One pediatric ICU study documented an average total sleep time of 4.7 hours, reduced 50% from baseline home sleep amounts, as well as decreased amounts of slow-wave sleep. These sleep disturbances may also persist after discharge, often as a result of learned associations and inadvertent parental reinforcement of maladaptive sleep patterns.

- **Medications.** Many of the medications used to treat children with a variety of medical problems are known to have potential adverse effects on sleep and/or to be associated with daytime sedation (see Chapter 19 for a more detailed discussion of pharmacologic effects on sleep). These include analgesics for pain management, antihistamines/antipruritics for allergies, bronchodilators and corticosteroids for asthma, various chemotherapeutic agents, and anticonvulsants for seizures.

Sleep and Quality of Life

Virtually any medical condition, acute or chronic, may have adverse effects on a child's sleep quality and quantity. Multiple possible contributing factors should be considered, including concomitant medications, psychosocial factors, and pain. Because of the potential impact of sleep disturbances on both the underlying disease process and the child's and family's quality of life, the practitioner should make every effort to assess for and address sleep problems in the setting of medical illness.

SPECIFIC MEDICAL CONDITIONS

Specific medical conditions that have been reported in association with poor quality and/or inadequate sleep are discussed below (medical conditions that are associated with significant developmental delay are included in Chapter 20). However, it should be noted that virtually every medical condition in children and adolescents, because of related issues such as stress, pain, and medication use, may be accompanied and exacerbated by disrupted sleep. For example, a primary cardiac or respiratory disease may result in sleep disturbances, and the underlying disease may be exacerbated during sleep. Medical disorders that affect the upper or lower respiratory system can result in sleep disruption. Any disorders that result in increased upper airway resistance, decreased functional residual volume, increased secretions in the airway, altered chest wall mechanics, abnormal central respiratory control, or underlying chronic lung disease can exacerbate sleep disordered breathing and cause sleep disruption.

(Note: Medical conditions are presented in alphabetical order, with seizures and central hypoventilation syndrome covered as separate sections at the end of the chapter.)

Allergies

Chronic allergy-mediated rhinitis with nasal congestion and cough, and chronic/frequent sinusitis are not only associated with difficulties initiating and maintaining sleep, but are also considered to be risk factors for obstructive sleep apnea and contribute to upper airway resistance. Use of sedating antihistamines to control allergic symptoms during the day may also disrupt regular sleep–wake patterns. Adequate nocturnal, as well as diurnal control of symptoms such as wheezing, cough, and pruritus, should be a primary goal in the management of atopic disease. This often requires the use of measures to control allergens in the sleeping environment (protective mattress and pillow covers, hypoallergenic bed clothes), as well as pharmacologic intervention.

Asthma

Asthma is known in adults to affect quality of sleep; in children it has been associated with poorer subjective sleep quality, decreased sleep duration, increased nocturnal wakings with decreased sleep efficiency, reduced slow-wave sleep, and greater daytime sleepiness. The underlying asthma symptoms may worsen at night as a result of circadian variations in respiratory function and peak flows and result in more disrupted sleep. Unlike normal children, patients with asthma, especially with suboptimal control, are likely to have more decreases in oxygen saturation compounding the disrupted sleep. In a number of studies, sleep symptoms have been correlated with subjective (symptoms) and objective (such as pulmonary function tests) measures of disease severity. The prevalence of sleep problems in children with asthma has been reported to be 60%. Nocturnal asthma symptoms (nighttime cough, frequent awakenings, etc.) have been associated in several studies with impaired daytime cognitive functioning, decreased school attendance and performance, and parental missed work. Cognitive function appears to improve with medication adjustment and optimal symptom control; however, some studies suggest that even children with well-controlled asthma may have more disrupted sleep than normal controls. Asthma also seems to be a separate risk factor for obstructive sleep apnea, further disrupting sleep and exacerbating daytime impairment.

Asthma medications may also have adverse effects on sleep; for example, oral corticosteroids may cause significant sleep disruption. Theophylline is known to have a stimulatory effect on the central nervous system (CNS) with resultant increased wakefulness, although in some studies it was not found to directly disrupt sleep. Theophylline may even exert a protective effect on apnea/hypopneas and oxygen saturation in the setting of sleep disordered breathing. "Insomnia" has been reported as an occasional side effect of leukotriene inhibitors; most of the newer asthma medications have more selective β-adrenergic and fewer CNS effects. In considering treatment options, it is important to weigh the benefits of good pharmacologic control against the possible negative effects of bronchodilators and other medications on sleep.

Atopic Dermatitis/Eczema

Atopic dermatitis may cause sleep disruption and fragmentation, difficulty falling asleep, night awakenings, and decreased sleep duration as a result of frequent scratching and discomfort. Parents of children with chronic allergies and/or atopic dermatitis may also be more aware of and pay more attention to nightwakings, further perpetuating the cycle of disrupted sleep.

Burns

Children who are severely burned are at particularly high risk for sleep problems, which, in turn, may have significant adverse effects on their recovery. Difficulty falling asleep, increased arousals, nightmares, and increased daytime sleepiness are common in the acute phase and may persist for up to a year after the event. Changes in sleep architecture have been reported, including decreased slow-wave sleep, which may contribute to the growth hormone insufficiency seen in burned children. It has been postulated that increases in particular types of peripheral cytokines in response to thermal injury (interleukin-1 and tumor necrosis factor) may contribute to sleep disruption through their specific role in sleep regulation. Burned children obviously also have multiple sources of pain, as well as severe pruritus, which may disrupt sleep. Additional factors are those common to all medically compromised and traumatized children, such as depression, anxiety/stress, posttraumatic stress disorder, and hospitalization/ICU-related factors. Narcotic analgesics, sedatives, and other medications used to treat anxiety (benzodiazepines) and depression in burned children may also alter sleep architecture.

Chronic Fatigue Syndrome

Chronic fatigue syndrome in adults and children has been reported to be associated with chronic sleep disturbances, including sleep onset and maintenance problems, and daytime sleepiness. These may further exacerbate symptoms of daytime fatigue.

Cystic Fibrosis

Decreased sleep efficiency and increased arousals and awakenings are common in children and adolescents with cystic fibrosis. Some awakenings are related to disease severity. Furthermore, nocturnal hypoxemia and oxygen desaturations during sleep are more common with progressive disease. There also appears to be an increased prevalence of sleep disordered breathing in cystic fibrosis. Nasal polyps and chronic sinusitis may further contribute to sleep disruption.

Fibromyalgia

Poor sleep is also part of the diagnostic criteria for juvenile fibromyalgia and may include prolonged sleep onset, frequent arousals, and decreased sleep efficiency, as well as periodic limb movements disrupting sleep. These sleep disturbances can potentially contribute to the daytime sleepiness/fatigue, depressed mood, and cognitive difficulties frequently associated with this painful musculoskeletal condition.

Gastrointestinal Disorders

Gastrointestinal disorders, especially those of a more chronic nature such as irritable bowel syndrome, have been associated with poor sleep quality in adults;

an underlying dysregulation mechanism resulting in both altered gastrointestinal function and sleep–wake regulation has been postulated. Chronic steroid use in inflammatory bowel disease may result in increased agitation at bedtime with sleep onset delay and increased hunger, leading to nocturnal eating.

Gastroesophageal Reflux Disease

Although studies have suggested that episodes of reflux are more likely to occur in the awake rather than the sleep (supine) state, episodes that do occur during sleep may be associated with prolonged clearance of acid from the esophagus and potentially the hypopharynx, with more severe mucosal damage. Chronic acid reflux is often associated with frequent arousals during sleep. In addition, gastroesophageal reflux disease (GERD) is associated with increased risk of aspiration, particularly in children with neurodevelopmental problems such as cerebral palsy. GERD may disrupt sleep because of secondary chronic cough and other respiratory symptoms as well as heartburn. GERD is also considered to be a risk factor for obstructive sleep apnea because of the associated mucosal edema. Furthermore, obstructive sleep apnea may exacerbate GERD and sleep disruption because the negative pressure generated to overcome the obstruction predisposes the patient to reflux. Anti-reflux medications that have serotonergic effects such as cisapride may also result in sleep disruption.

Juvenile Rheumatoid Arthritis

As noted above, any chronic medical condition that is characterized by recurrent pain may be associated with sleep disruption. Children with juvenile rheumatoid arthritis have been shown to have more frequent nightwakings and sleep fragmentation that may be associated with daytime sleepiness. At least in some studies, these sleep disruptions have been correlated with both pain and disease activity, suggesting the potential benefits of aggressive nocturnal pain management. The etiology of sleep problems in juvenile rheumatoid arthritis is likely multifactorial and may also include an increased prevalence of primary sleep disorders such as restless legs syndrome (see Chapter 14), periodic limb movement disorder (see Chapter 14), and obstructive sleep apnea (see Chapter 13).

Migraines

Migraine headaches have been associated with sleep onset and maintenance problems, as well as with an increased incidence of sleepwalking. Furthermore, sleep deprivation may trigger headaches in susceptible individuals. More sleep problems have been reported to occur with tension headaches as well, and may be related to increased stress and anxiety. Rebound headache pain related to frequent use of analgesic medications may be a contributing factor in some children.

Meningomyelocele

Meningomyelocele, especially when accompanied by type II Arnold-Chiari malformation, may result in a blunted respiratory drive during sleep with central apneas and may result in an increased risk for upper airway obstruction. Patients with thoracic or lumbar lesions are at increased risk for sleep disordered breathing, which may result in sleep disturbance. Patients with restrictive lung disease, such as wheel-chair-dependent patients with scoliosis, are also at increased risk for sleep disordered breathing.

Neuromuscular Disorders

Sleep disordered breathing and upper airway obstruction are more common in children with a variety of neuromuscular conditions, including Duchenne muscular dystrophy, Charcot-Marie-Tooth disease, myotonic dystrophy, and congenital myopathies characterized by hypotonia. In some of these conditions, the sleep disordered breathing is a result of respiratory muscle weakness and in others is related to reduced central ventilatory drive. The risk of respiratory desaturations or hypoxemia is greatest during REM sleep. Many of these children also have reduced vital capacity associated with scoliosis, which may further compromise respiratory function and exacerbate sleep disordered breathing. Many of these patients do not report obstructive sleep apnea–associated symptoms (e.g., snoring, daytime sleepiness, morning headaches) unless specifically asked, so that frequent screening for sleep disordered breathing symptoms is mandatory.

Increased risk for respiratory failure also is associated with generalized or proximal muscle weakness in these children, particularly those with diaphragmatic involvement and those who have had an earlier age of onset of symptoms. Significant sleep disordered breathing can occur in the setting of even mild respiratory muscle weakness. The hypoxemia and chronic respiratory failure in these patients is usually preceded by periods of increased end-tidal CO_2 during sleep. Daytime blood gases may be normal. Pulmonary function tests are often noncontributory but may show restrictive lung disease, and there may be minimal symptoms of sleep disordered breathing. Furthermore, pulmonary function testing to assess maximal inspiratory and expiratory pressures can he helpful to assess the severity of muscle weakness.

Sleep and Neurologic Disorders

The primary care practitioner should maintain a high level of suspicion for sleep disordered breathing, particularly in children with neuromuscular disorders and spina bifida, as this may be overlooked in the context of multiple other medical needs. Close collaboration with a multidisciplinary neuro-rehabilitation team for follow-up is strongly recommended.

Phenylketonuria

Phenylketonuria may be associated with difficulties in sleep onset and maintenance, as well as nightmares related to an increase in the amount of REM sleep. These sleep disturbances may be a result of alterations in the phenylalanine/tyrosine/tryptophan ratio. A balanced phenylalanine-restricted diet may be helpful in reducing sleep disruption.

Chronic Renal Failure

Sleep disruption in children with chronic renal failure may be related to a number of factors, including medications, dialysis, or decreased urine output. There is an increased prevalence of restless legs syndrome and periodic limb movement disorder (see Chapter 14) in chronic renal failure, which may lead to delayed sleep onset, fragmented sleep, and excessive daytime sleepiness. Increased daytime somnolence may also be a result of increasing renal failure.

Sickle Cell Disease

Painful nocturnal crises and direct and indirect effects of analgesics, including opiates, may clearly impact on sleep patterns in children with sickle cell disease. These children may also be prone to sleep disordered breathing as a result of adenotonsillar hypertrophy related to compensatory lymphoid hyperplasia with functional asplenia, repeated infections, and airway narrowing related to the anatomic effects of bone marrow hyperplasia. Hypoxemia related to obstructive sleep apnea may lead to increased nocturnal sickling and pain crises with resultant exacerbation of the disease. Some authors suggest that daytime oxyhemoglobin saturation may be a better predictor of nocturnal hypoxemia associated with obstructive sleep apnea in these children than history and physical findings. Hypoxemia may significantly improve with adenotonsillectomy, although clearly these children are at higher surgical risk for perioperative complications as a result of their disease.

Traumatic Brain Injury

Changes occurring in sleep architecture during the acute phase following head injury electroencephalography include increased slow-wave sleep. A postconcussive syndrome and/or posttraumatic stress disorder symptoms with resultant difficulties in sleep initiation and maintenance, early morning waking, decreased sleep quality, and daytime sleepiness have been reported with even relatively minor head injuries. These sleep abnormalities may persist for several years.

SLEEP AND SEIZURE DISORDERS

Although a detailed description of the complex interaction between epilepsy and sleep is beyond the scope of this book, a number of important points relevant to the primary care physician must be mentioned. It is estimated that 20% to 40% of seizures in childhood occur during sleep; some types of seizures, such as benign rolandic epilepsy and frontal lobe seizures, occur primarily or exclusively during sleep. Childhood seizures are especially prominent in sleep stages 1 and 2, although a significant percentage also occur at the sleep–wake transition (e.g., infantile spasms, some tonic-clonic seizures). In general, seizures are uncommon during other sleep stages such as slow-wave sleep, although partial complex seizures may occur solely in REM sleep. In one study, about half of first-time unprovoked seizures occurred during sleep. Furthermore, the likelihood of recurrence was significantly increased (42% versus 18%) in those children who presented with nocturnal seizures.

Seizures and Sleep

In contrast to adults, nocturnal seizures are quite common in children, and some types of seizures (e.g., those of benign rolandic epilepsy) occur predominantly during sleep. Nocturnal seizures may cause significant sleep disruption and daytime sleepiness. Alternatively, sleep deprivation is a well-established trigger factor for seizures. Nocturnal seizures are more common in non-REM sleep, and it is postulated that seizures may be triggered by or during the intrinsic rhythmicity of these non-REM stages (primarily stage 2).

Seizures (including rolandic epilepsy, tonic-clonic) may cause sleep disruption, and there is a higher incidence of sleep disturbances in patients with epilepsy in general. Seizure activity does not need to be overt to disrupt sleep but rather may consist of brief stereotypic arousals and microarousals that result in significant daytime sleepiness. Successful anticonvulsant therapy may alleviate daytime somnolence even in the absence of frank seizure activity, although anticonvulsants may clearly cause sedation as well. Neurodevelopmental disorders (e.g., severe developmental delay, blindness) that are frequently associated with seizures as part of their clinical presentation may also predispose the patient to sleep disorders. Sleep disorders may also exacerbate seizures in patients with known epilepsy. For example, hypoxia and sleep fragmentation associated with obstructive sleep apnea may trigger seizures in a predisposed child, as may any sleep disorder associated with significant sleep deprivation. However, it should be kept in mind that the limited electroencephalographic montage used in most overnight sleep studies to determine sleep stages may be inadequate to detect many types of seizures.

The role of sleep deprivation as a well-known trigger for seizures also may assist in the diagnostic process. Relative sleep deprivation may increase electroencephalographic abnormalities by three- to fourfold; as many as one-third of patients with clinical seizures and normal/borderline electroencephalograms (EEGs) show abnormal discharges after sleep deprivation, and up to half of patients may show additional epileptiform features compared to the non-sleep-deprived EEG. A sleep-deprived EEG may be considered when seizures are strongly suspected on clinical grounds; routine electroencephalography does not reveal definite abnormalities, and should include partial sleep deprivation (delayed bedtime and early waketime) in children, and nap deprivation in infants/toddlers.

Sleep Studies and Seizures

Because not all sleep laboratories perform a full electroencephalographic seizure montage as part of routine polysomnography, an overnight sleep study alone may not be sufficient to rule out nocturnal seizures. Additional diagnostic procedures, such as 24-hour ambulatory electroencephalographic monitoring, may be necessary in cases in which there is a high index of suspicion.

Nocturnal seizures may be difficult to distinguish from other episodic nocturnal phenomena, including partial arousal parasomnias (see Chapter 10 for complete coverage of differentiating seizures from parasomnias). Parasomnias may also occur in children with known seizure disorders. Frontal lobe seizures may have similar clinical presentation as parasomnias, with a normal baseline neurologic exam and a normal EEG even during the event (given the limitations of surface electroencephalographic recordings). Postictal events (e.g., confusion, weakness), as reported by the patient or observer, are more difficult to establish in nocturnal seizures. Differential diagnoses also include other primary sleep disorders: bruxism, rhythmic movement disorders, nocturnal myoclonus and sleep starts, periodic limb movements, obstructive sleep apnea, REM behavior disorder (extremely rare in childhood and only reported in the setting of CNS pathology), enuresis, hynogogic hallucinations and sleep paralysis associated with narcolepsy; nocturnal physiologic arousals related to medical conditions (e.g., GERD, asthma); psychiatric disorders (nocturnal panic attacks, posttraumatic stress disorder), and psychogenic seizures.

Specific sleep-related epilepsies include:

- **Benign rolandic epilepsy** is a common, autosomal dominant form of epilepsy, accounting for about 15% of childhood epilepsies. The onset is usually in middle childhood. Seizures are usually limited to sleep, are focal in nature, generally involve the face/upper extremities with associated speech arrest, and are frequently described as tingling, twitching, and/or numbness by the patient who is awake and aware of the sensations. Seizures may occasionally spread to generalized tonic-clonic activity. These children have normal sleep organization with a central/midtemporal focus that is increased by sleepiness. The prognosis for resolution of seizures, as the name implies, is excellent, and anticonvulsant therapy may not be indicated.

- **Infantile spasms** frequently have their onset in the first 4 to 7 months of life and are characterized by abrupt spasms, extension of the arms/legs, and flexion at the waist, occurring in clusters at the sleep–wake transition or shortly after awakening. The EEG shows the characteristic hypsarrhythmia pattern of high-voltage spikes and disorganized background. Patients with infantile spasms can be difficult to treat, but may respond to pharmacologic therapy or hormonal therapy (adrenocorticotropic hormone). These patients are at risk for severe developmental delay.

- **Nocturnal paroxysmal dystonias** are characterized by sustained dystonic posturing of the trunk and extremities in non-REM sleep with immediate return to sleep after seconds to several minutes. Patients with nocturnal paroxysmal dystonia may have nocturnal frontal lobe epilepsy and may respond to carbamazepine.

- **Juvenile myoclonic epilepsy** is probably an autosomal dominant epilepsy that presents in adolescence and is characterized by myoclonic activity (jerking of the arms and often the legs). Alcohol, stress, sleep deprivation, and flickering lights may exacerbate seizure activity. In addition, patients may have other types of seizures (e.g., absence seizures, atonic spells, generalized tonic-clonic seizures).

Finally, anticonvulsants may compromise the sleep–wake cycle by causing daytime sedation and increasing the frequency of those types of seizures that are exacerbated by sleepiness (like absence), whereas other anticonvulsants have been associated with prolonged sleep onset and arousals. Anticonvulsant withdrawal can also result in sleep difficulties, especially with GABAergic medications like benzodiazepines. Anticonvulsants associated with decreased REM sleep, such as barbiturates, may lead to REM rebound (increased nightmares) on withdrawal. Oftentimes, however, appropriate treatment with anticonvulsants to eliminate or reduce nocturnal seizure activity actually improves sleep by decreasing sleep onset time and nighttime arousals.

CENTRAL HYPOVENTILATION SYNDROMES

Defective autonomic control of breathing may occur in association with medical conditions such as Hirschsprung disease, inborn errors of metabolism and neuroblastoma, or in a congenital form [idiopathic congenital central hypoventilation syndrome (CCHS)]. CCHS is a rare disorder, with likely fewer than 300 living children worldwide. It typically presents in the newborn period with symptoms including duskiness or cyanosis upon falling asleep, and decreasing oxygen saturation with hypercarbia and hypoventilation during sleep. Because of the lack or reduction of ventilatory sensitivity to hypoxemia and hypercarbia, children with CCHS do not have an arousal response or behavioral awareness of asphyxia. Prompt referral and evaluation is warranted for children with persistent hypoxemia or hypercarbia or abnormal gas exchange even in the absence of respiratory or neurocognitive symptoms.

TREATMENT

Management of sleep problems in children with acute and chronic medical conditions first requires recognition on the part of the practitioner of the existence of possible risk factors for sleep disturbances and the high likelihood of their occurrence, particularly in some disease states and in certain settings, as outlined above. Symptoms such as fatigue, mood changes, and particularly daytime sleepiness in chronically ill children should not be automatically attributed to the underlying disease process, and every effort should be made to screen for and address primary and secondary sleep problems when they occur. Medication choices should take into consideration any possible negative effects on sleep. In addition, those pain medications likely to disrupt sleep or significantly alter sleep architecture, such as opiates and benzodiazepines, should be avoided or used for short time intervals. In contrast, nonsteroidal antiinflammatory and nonopiate analgesics, especially when used in the short term, have little overall effect on sleep.

Approaches to pain management in children that may have particularly beneficial effects on sleep as well include:

- Use of relaxation techniques, including hypnosis and biofeedback.
- Incorporation of cognitive behavioral therapy aimed at management of chronic pain and development of age-appropriate and adaptive coping skills.
- Support of parent education and modeling of good sleep habits.
- Maintenance of regular daytime and particularly bedtime routines.

Consultation for Sleep Issues

Children with chronic medical conditions and sleep issues, and hospitalized children in particular, often benefit from consultation with a child life specialist and/or behavioral therapist regarding specific management strategies. Additional input from a consultation-liaison child psychiatry team may be beneficial if pharmacologic intervention is being considered.

In children who are hospitalized, attention should be paid to the possible sleep-disrupting effects of the hospital environment, and every effort should be made to minimize nighttime interruptions, such as noise, lights, and stimulation (e.g., television), maintain structured bedtimes and routines, and avoid inappropriate sleep associations. For example, some studies suggest that parental presence and reminders of home may actually exacerbate sleep problems, but clearly this varies across individual children at different developmental stages.

Any child with a medical condition that may pose an increased risk for sleep disordered breathing (e.g., neuromuscular disorders, chronic allergies) should be monitored regularly for the development of possible signs and symptoms, such as snoring, restless sleep, and daytime sleepiness. A high index of suspicion and a low threshold for obtaining an overnight sleep study evaluation is particularly important in these children. Ongoing consultation with a pediatric sleep specialist and/or pulmonologist is recommended.

22

Sleep and Psychiatric Disorders

GENERAL CONSIDERATIONS

Sleep disturbances are highly prevalent in children and adolescents with psychiatric disorders. Primary behavioral and psychiatric disorders in children are frequently associated with and/or complicated by sleep problems, which may be related to such factors as the psychopathology of the underlying disorder, comorbid conditions, or pharmacologic treatment. Conversely, neurobehavioral symptoms, ranging from mood lability to attentional problems to school failure, are common primary presenting symptoms for both intrinsic (e.g., obstructive sleep apnea) and extrinsic sleep disorders (those related to environmental factors, such as parental limit setting).

Several studies have evaluated the prevalence of sleep problems in samples of children and adolescents with a variety of psychiatric disorders. These studies suggest that there is an increase in a wide range of reported sleep disturbances in these clinical populations, including difficulty falling asleep; frequent and prolonged nightwakings; sleep-related anxiety symptoms (e.g., fear of the dark); restless sleep; parasomnias (e.g., nightmares, night terrors); subjective poor quality of sleep; and daytime fatigue. Similarly, an association has been reported between psychiatric disorders, including mood disorders and conduct disorders, and sleep problems in surveys of children and adolescents from the general population.

Given the prevalence of sleep problems in association with psychiatric conditions, it is important to evaluate and treat sleep disturbances in all children presenting with psychiatric, behavioral, and academic concerns. The most common psychiatric disorders in childhood for which we have information regarding the relationship between sleep and psychiatric symptoms are highlighted.

Sleep and Neurobehavioral Symptoms: A Bidirectional Relationship

There is clearly a bidirectional relationship between sleep, mood, and behavior in childhood. Inadequate sleep often results in neurobehavioral symptoms, including mood disturbances, cognitive impairment, inattentiveness, and behavior problems. Conversely, children with mood and behavior disorders often experience sleep disturbances.

ATTENTION DEFICIT-HYPERACTIVITY DISORDER

General Description

Many children and adolescents who have been diagnosed with attention deficit-hyperactivity disorder (ADHD; hyperactive/impulsive, inattentive, and combined subtypes) have sleep problems. Parents frequently complain of bedtime struggles and delayed sleep onset, increased nightwakings, restless sleep, and shortened sleep duration in these children. In general, studies using more "objective" means of assessing sleep quality and quantity, such as polysomnography and actigraphy (a wristwatch-like device that measures sleep/wake periods), do not support consistent differences in sleep patterns and sleep architecture between children with ADHD and normal controls. This discrepancy between parental reports and objective findings may be in part due to the important influence of two factors commonly associated with ADHD: comorbid psychiatric conditions and the use of medications to treat ADHD that may have effects on sleep (e.g., stimulants such as methylphenidate and dextroamphetamine).

The relationship between sleep disturbance and ADHD is further complicated by the considerable overlap between many of the most common behavioral consequences of inadequate or disrupted sleep in children and the symptoms of ADHD. These include problems with attention and focusing, hyperactivity, irritability and disturbed mood, and "acting out" behaviors characterized by increased aggression and poor impulse control.

Recent research has begun to document that a percentage of children (mis)diagnosed with primary ADHD actually have a primary sleep disorder, including obstructive sleep apnea, restless legs syndrome, and periodic limb movement disorder. Studies suggest that snoring is about one and a half times more frequent in children with hyperactivity and that, in turn, between 10% and 15% of children with academic problems have symptoms of obstructive sleep apnea. It has been estimated that up to 25% of children with ADHD may have significant sleep disordered breathing. In another study, more than half of children evaluated for ADHD in a pediatric neurology clinic were found to have clinical and polysomnographic evidence of restless legs syndrome and/or periodic limb movement disorder (see Chapter 14). Furthermore, sleep disorders add to the severity of ADHD symptoms when they coexist. Thus, all children with ADHD should be periodically screened for sleep disturbances.

Sleep Disorders and ADHD

The relationship between sleep disturbances and ADHD is a complex and multifactorial one. Sleep problems in these children may be related to hyperarousal intrinsic to the ADHD, comorbid psychiatric conditions, concomitant medications (especially psychostimulants), and/or coexisting primary sleep disorders. A thorough search for possible etiologic factors is necessary in order to develop the most appropriate treatment plan.

Epidemiology

Despite the fact that studies, in general, do not support the existence of an "intrinsic" sleep disorder in children with ADHD, pediatricians are often confronted with the child with ADHD who "won't sleep." The prevalence of parent-reported sleep problems in ADHD has been reported to be as high as 50% to 60% with bedtime resistance/sleep onset delay and 50% to 60% with restless sleep.

Etiology

Because the etiology of sleep problems in children with ADHD is so varied and often multifactorial, considerable care should be taken to examine the following possible causes:

- **A primary sleep disorder may result in "ADHD"-like symptoms.** Any sleep disorder that results in inadequate sleep duration, fragmented/disrupted sleep, or excessive daytime sleepiness may cause problems with mood, attention, and behavior. For example, obstructive sleep apnea may be associated with behavioral symptoms such as inattentiveness and distractibility, hyperactivity, and poor impulse control. Furthermore, these symptoms may be improved or even eliminated with treatment of the obstructive sleep apnea (e.g., adenotonsillectomy). Restless legs syndrome/periodic limb movement disorder, delayed sleep phase, and narcolepsy are other specific sleep disorders that have been reported in association with ADHD symptoms.
- **Coexisting sleep disturbances may exacerbate the symptoms of ADHD.** Sleep disorders such as obstructive sleep apnea may occur in conjunction with ADHD, and the cognitive, mood, and behavioral disturbances associated with ADHD may be worsened by the presence of these sleep disorders.

Inadequate sleep related to environmental or lifestyle factors (e.g., erratic schedules), particularly if chronic, may exacerbate ADHD symptoms. Some children with ADHD, especially older children, may have a delayed sleep phase, which may contribute to difficulties settling at bedtime and prolonged sleep onset. Treatment of comorbid sleep disorders and interventions targeted at ensuring adequate sleep may substantially improve daytime ADHD symptoms.

- **Coexisting psychiatric disorders may be the underlying cause of sleep disturbance in a child with ADHD.** Many children with ADHD have other psychiatric disorders in addition to ADHD, such as oppositional defiant disorder, anxiety and mood disorders, and Tourette syndrome, that may contribute to sleep problems. For example, limit setting problems associated with ODD may result in bedtime resistance, whereas depression and anxiety may be associated with difficulties falling and staying asleep. Fifty percent of Tourette syndrome patients have been reported to have sleep disturbances, including enuresis and partial arousal parasomnias, such as sleepwalking. Furthermore, motor tics associated with Tourette syndrome may occur during sleep, resulting in sleep fragmentation. Pharmacologic treatment of the tics (e.g., clonidine, clonezepam) may improve sleep quality in these patients. Problems with sensory integration and associated difficulties in self-soothing may also predispose children with ADHD to sleep onset and settling problems.

- **Pharmacologic agents used to treat ADHD and/or comorbid psychiatric conditions may cause or exacerbate sleep problems.** In particular, psychostimulant medication may be associated with sleep onset and maintenance problems and restless sleep. Sleep problems may be a direct effect of the medication itself, and thus dosage or dosing schedule adjustments or alternative treatment with nonstimulants may be beneficial. In other cases, stimulant medication may wear off just before bedtime, resulting in "rebound" hyperactivity and, indirectly, sleep onset difficulties. In this situation, an additional late-day dose of stimulant medication that lasts through bedtime may be helpful in some cases. Alpha agonists are also widely used to address stimulant-induced insomnia (see section "Treatment" below). Newer, nonstimulant medications for ADHD, such as atomoxetine, may have relatively fewer sleep-related side effects. Finally, other psychiatric medications used in children with ADHD, including different classes of antidepressants (see Chapter 19), may also cause sleep problems.

- **Poor CNS regulation of arousal/activity associated with ADHD may result in sleep disturbances.** Although the presence of an "intrinsic" dysfunction linking sleep disturbances and ADHD is largely speculative at this point, difficulties in "settling" or "turning off" at bedtime are commonly reported in children with ADHD. Significant problems with delayed sleep onset appear to occur in these children in the absence of other identifiable causes, such as use of medication.

Risk Factors

In addition to use of stimulant medications and comorbid psychiatric disorders, risk factors for sleep disturbances in ADHD appear to include younger age and hyperactive/impulsive subtype of ADHD. Furthermore, ADHD children who snore may be at particular risk for primary or coexisting sleep disordered breathing.

Evaluation

- **Screening for sleep disorders should be part of the evaluation for every child with suspected ADHD.** Screening questions regarding sleep onset, nightwakings, restless sleep, snoring, sleep regularity and duration, and day-time sleepiness should be part of every ADHD evaluation. Sleep diaries may be very helpful in identifying problem sleep patterns and behaviors. Clinical suspicion of a sleep disorder warrants appropriate diagnostic evaluation, such as an overnight sleep study to evaluate for obstructive sleep apnea.
- **Periodic screening for sleep disorders should be part of the ongoing management of every child with diagnosed ADHD.** Comorbid psychiatric conditions and associated sleep problems may evolve in children with ADHD. Changes in medication type, dose, and dosing schedule over the course of treatment may result in sleep disturbances. Comorbid sleep problems, such as obstructive sleep apnea, may also develop over time, especially in high-risk groups such as obese children.

Screening for Sleep Disorders (BEARS)

- **B:** Does your child have any problems going to **B**ed or any problems falling asleep?
- **E:** Does your child show symptoms of **E**xcessive daytime sleepiness (seem sleepy during the day and/or have difficulty waking up in the morning)?
- **A:** Does your child **A**waken during the night or have any unusual behaviors during the night?
- **R:** Does your child have a **R**egular sleep schedule and get enough sleep?
- **S:** Does your child **S**nore or have any problems breathing during the night?

Treatment

- **Etiologically-based intervention.** Treatment for sleep disturbances in ADHD should be matched to the underlying etiology in each individual case. Thus, if sleep disordered breathing (see Chapter 13) or periodic limb movement disorder (see Chapter 14) is felt to play an etiologic or exacerbating role regarding

ADHD symptoms, management should be directed toward treating the primary sleep disorder. In the case of psychiatric conditions, antidepressant or antianxiety medications may alleviate associated sleep problems but care should be taken to avoid pharmacologic agents that may exacerbate sleep disturbances. Behavioral interventions targeted at relieving anxiety (e.g., relaxation techniques) or addressing oppositional behaviors (e.g., positive reinforcement, ignoring) should be included and may require the assistance of a behavioral consultant. Adjustments in the types, dose, and dosing schedules of ADHD medications may be warranted if these are suspected of contributing to the sleep problems.

• **Pharmacologic interventions.** Some children with severe sleep onset problems that are not due to other underlying conditions may benefit from pharmacologic intervention at bedtime in conjunction with good sleep hygiene and behavioral management. A medication that is commonly prescribed in this situation is the α agonist clonidine. Clonidine, originally developed as an antihypertensive medication, is used to treat daytime symptoms of hyperactivity and impulsivity in ADHD; however, sedation effects and short half-life, two properties that add to its utility as a sleep medication, often limit its use. A small dose (ranging from 0.025 or one fourth of a 0.1-mg tablet in younger children up to a maximum of 0.3 mg in adolescents) 30 minutes before lights out may be helpful in inducing sleep onset. Because of potential cardiac conduction effects, the practitioner should consider obtaining an electrocardiogram at baseline and after initiation of treatment, particularly if clonidine is given in combination with a psychostimulant. Blood pressure should be monitored during treatment. Abrupt discontinuation of clonidine may be associated with rebound hypertension; therefore, parents should be cautioned against stopping medication suddenly. Some minor anticholinergic effects (dry mouth, constipation) are occasionally seen. Children may develop a tolerance to the dose and require periodic increases.

MOOD DISORDERS

General Description

The interaction between sleep disturbances and symptoms of mood dysregulation such as anxiety and depression may pose a diagnostic dilemma because of the overlap in symptoms between the two. Studies of mixed clinical psychiatric populations, for example, have suggested that 40% to 50% of these children have parent-reported nightwakings, nightmares, and difficulty waking in the morning. In addition, there may be therapeutic challenges in setting treatment priorities regarding interventions for mood disorders; for example, pharmacotherapy for a mood disorder may cause sleep disruption and result in worsening of the mood problems. At the very least, the consequences of disrupted or inadequate sleep may exacerbate mood disorders, which, in turn, may lead to additional sleep disturbances in a negative spiral.

Specific Disorders

Depression

Although electroencephalographic sleep changes, particularly decreased latency to REM sleep onset, have been clearly shown to be a marker for adult depression, these abnormalities have not been consistently found in depressed children and adolescents. However, a number of studies, as well as clinical experience, have suggested that significant difficulty in falling asleep is commonly associated with childhood depression (including major depressive disorder and dysthymia) and may in fact predict future mood disturbances in adulthood. Subjective poor sleep quality and sleep–wake cycle irregularities are also common. Hypersomnia, or excessive sleep, is sometimes associated with childhood depression, occurring in as much as 25% of depressed adolescents. Many antidepressants, most notably the selective serotonin reuptake inhibitors (SSRIs), have sleep disruptive effects or may cause daytime sedation (see Chapter 19 for more information on the effects of medication on sleep).

Bipolar Disorder

Bipolar disorder has been increasingly recognized in the past decade as a potential cause of severe behavioral and emotional disturbances in childhood and adolescence. Particularly in its earliest stages, the symptoms of marked and frequent mood swings, explosive outbursts, and extreme defiance may be labeled as ADHD or oppositional defiant disorder. Children with bipolar disorder often have sleep problems, ranging from difficulty waking in the morning to intense nightmares. They may exhibit a sleep phase delay pattern with decreased alertness in the morning and increasing levels of energy and mood intensity late in the day, leading to bedtime struggles. In some patients, this alteration in circadian timing appears to be exaggerated by seasonal changes in ambient light, and thus may be responsive to bright light phototherapy. Studies have also demonstrated that even one night of sleep deprivation may trigger a switch into a manic or hypomanic episode. Sleep needs may also be significantly decreased in the manic phase in adolescents with bipolar disorder, and a period of increasingly shorter sleep intervals may herald the onset of a manic episode. Finally, medications used to treat bipolar disorder may result in sleep disruption or daytime sedation (e.g., valproic acid, risperidone).

Anxiety Disorders

Sleep disturbances are also commonly experienced in relation to childhood and adolescent anxiety disorders.

- **Adjustment disorders.** Sleep problems are frequently associated with adjustment disorders, which are reactions to minor stressful life events such as brief separation from a parent, birth of a sibling, or school transitions. These sleep problems, which frequently include bedtime resistance and nightwakings, may immediately follow the stressful event or may have a more gradual onset. Delayed sleep onset is often characterized by clinginess and refusal to be separated from the caregiver in younger children, and rumination and "free-floating" anxiety in the older child. Parents may prolong adjustment sleep problems by inadvertently providing continued reinforcement (attention) for bedtime resistance, even after the original anxiety symptoms have been alleviated.

- **Nighttime fears.** Nighttime fears, which are often a reflection of normal developmental processes, are also extremely common especially in young children, and may lead to significant bedtime resistance and problematic nightwakings. It is important to distinguish between developmentally appropriate, nighttime anxiety–related behaviors and sleep-disrupting fears associated with more global daytime anxiety symptoms. The former is usually time limited, whereas the latter may be indicative of an anxiety disorder. If it is a more global anxiety disorder, the cognitive-behavioral techniques (positive reinforcement, self-control procedures, graduated extinction) often used successfully to treat isolated nighttime fears may be ineffective and more intensive intervention strategies (psychotherapy, anxiolytics) may be warranted.

- **Separation anxiety and generalized anxiety disorder.** Children with anxiety symptoms at bedtime may also have a more global and serious anxiety disorder, such as separation anxiety disorder and generalized anxiety disorder; these children frequently experience an exacerbation of symptoms at night. The degree, duration, and pervasiveness of the anxiety symptoms, as well as a family history of anxiety and mood disorders, may help to differentiate the child with more transient and situational nighttime anxiety from one with more chronic symptoms.

- **Posttraumatic stress disorder (PTSD).** Reports of sleep complaints, especially bedtime resistance, refusal to sleep alone, increased nighttime fears, and nightmares, are common in children with posttraumatic stress disorder who have experienced severely traumatic events (including physical and sexual abuse).

Sleep and Anxiety

Difficulties in initiating and maintaining sleep are often related to acute and/or chronic anxiety. In older children and adolescents in particular, it is important to differentiate between more transient, situational, and circumscribed nighttime anxiety, and sleep symptoms associated with more global daytime anxiety. The approach to treatment and the need for additional counseling and psychopharmacology in these two situations are often quite different.

Epidemiology

Sleep disturbances, especially "insomnia" (usually defined as difficulty initiating and/or maintaining sleep), are reported in up to 90% of children and adolescents with depression and anxiety disorders. For example, studies of children with major depressive disorder have reported that up to 75% meet the diagnostic criteria for insomnia and 30% for severe insomnia, although it should be noted that objective data (e.g., polysomnography) do not always support these subjective complaints.

Risk Factors

The presence of secondary factors, particularly in adolescence, such as alcohol use, cigarette smoking, substance abuse, and erratic sleep–wake schedules, may further predispose the depressed or anxious patient to sleep problems. The presence of comorbid psychiatric conditions and use of psychotropic medication are also likely to increase the risk for sleep disturbances in these patients.

Evaluation

Similar to adults, it is often difficult from a clinical standpoint to clearly distinguish between primary and secondary sleep disorders in children with behavioral and emotional problems. Therefore, it is incumbent on health care providers to evaluate and appropriately treat both because improvement in one is likely to have a positive impact on the related condition. Screening for sleep disorders should be part of the psychiatric evaluation for every child with mood or behavior problems. Furthermore, periodic screening for sleep disorders should be part of the ongoing management of every child with diagnosed psychiatric disorders, especially depression and anxiety.

Treatment

Integrated Treatment Approaches

Because of the frequent coexistence and bidirectional effects of sleep disturbances and mood/anxiety disorders, the most effective treatment approach generally involves addressing both concerns simultaneously. At the very least, care should be taken to avoid treatment strategies that may exacerbate comorbid sleep problems (e.g., antidepressants that have disruptive effects on sleep).

The goals of treating sleep problems in the context of mood and anxiety disorders should include:

- **Development of strategies to optimize regular and adequate sleep.** Setting a temporary later bedtime that coincides more closely with the actual sleep onset time may relieve some of the anxiety associated with trying to fall asleep. Bedtime strategies may be negotiated initially with the child, but once established should be consistently and firmly enforced to avoid inadvertent reinforcement of stalling behaviors.
- **Treatment of the primary psychiatric disorder** with psychotherapy and pharmacologic agents that do not exacerbate sleep disturbances. Because of the sleep-disrupting effects of some antidepressant medications (including SSRIs, venlafaxine, and bupropion), treatment of the underlying depression may actually exacerbate the sleep disturbance, so care should be taken.
- **Identification and elimination of additional factors** (e.g., alcohol use) that may be impacting on both the psychiatric disorder and the sleep disturbance.
- **Treatment of the associated sleep problems,** as there is usually some resulting degree of improvement in mood and fatigue. In cases of severe anxiety, the primary goal is reduction of the anxiety symptoms at bedtime, including use of gradual desensitization, bedtime checks, and gradual weaning of parental presence.
- **Institution of environmental changes,** such as nightlights or a fish tank in the child's bedroom, to relieve anxiety symptoms that occur at bedtime and throughout the night.
- **Teaching of relaxation technique,** such as deep breathing and visual imagery, that may help children to develop a sense of control over anxiety symptoms.
- **Referral for mental health counseling** in cases of severe anxiety or if mood symptoms are persistent and affect daytime functioning.

Appendix A

Sleep Evaluation Questionnaire

Sleep Evaluation Questionnaire

ID #

Directions

Please answer each of the following questions by writing in or choosing the best answer. This will help us know more about your family and your child.

CHILD'S INFORMATION	
Child's name:	Child's gender: ☐ Male ☐ Female
Child's birthdate:	Child's age:
Child's racial/ethnic background:	☐ White/Caucasian ☐ Black/African-American ☐ Asian-American ☐ Native-American ☐ Hispanic-Latino ☐ Multi-racial ☐ Other

What are your major concerns about your child's sleep?

What things have you tried to help your child's problem?

SLEEP HISTORY

Weekday Sleep Schedule

Write in the amount of time child sleeps during a 24-hour period <u>on weekdays</u> (add daytime and nighttime sleep):   _____ hours _____ minutes

The child's usual <u>bedtime</u> on <u>weekday nights</u> :   _____ : _____

The child's usual <u>waketime</u> on <u>weekday mornings</u>:   _____ : _____

Weekend/Vacation Sleep Schedule

Write in the amount of time child sleeps during a 24-hour period <u>during weekends and vacations</u> (add daytime and nighttime sleep):   _____ hours _____ minutes

The child's usual <u>bedtime</u> on <u>weekend/vacation nights</u> :   _____ : _____

The child's usual <u>waketime</u> on <u>weekend/vacation mornings</u>:   _____ : _____

Nap Schedule

Number of <u>days each week</u> child takes a nap: ☐ 0   ☐ 1   ☐ 2   ☐ 3   ☐ 4   ☐ 5   ☐ 6   ☐ 7

If child naps, write in usual nap time(S):   Nap 1:   ____ : ____   ☐ a.m. ☐ p.m. to ____ : ____   ☐ a.m. ☐ p.m.

Nap 2:   ____ : ____   ☐ a.m. ☐ p.m. to ____ : ____   ☐ a.m. ☐ p.m.

General Sleep

Does the child have a regular bedtime routine?	☐ yes ☐ no
Does the child have his/her own bedroom?	☐ yes ☐ no
Does the child have his/her own bed?	☐ yes ☐ no
Is a parent present when your child falls asleep?	☐ yes ☐ no

Child usually <u>falls asleep</u> in…	Child <u>sleeps most of the night</u> in…	Child usually <u>wakes in the morning</u> in…
☐ own room in own bed (alone)	☐ own room in own bed (alone)	☐ own room in own bed (alone)
☐ parents' room in own bed	☐ parents' room in own bed	☐ parents' room in own bed
☐ parents' room in parents' bed	☐ parents' room in parents' bed	☐ parents' room in parents' bed
☐ sibling's room in own bed	☐ sibling's room in own bed	☐ sibling's room in own bed
☐ sibling's room in sibling's bed	☐ sibling's room in sibling's bed	☐ sibling's room in sibling's bed

Child is usually put to bed by: ☐ Mother   ☐ Father   ☐ Both Parents   ☐ Self   ☐ Others

Write in the <u>amount of time</u> the child spends in <u>his/her bedroom</u> before going to sleep: _____ minutes

Child resists going to bed?	☐ yes ☐ no	**If yes,** do you think this is a problem?	☐ yes ☐ no
Child has difficulty falling asleep?	☐ yes ☐ no	**If yes,** do you think this is a problem?	☐ yes ☐ no
Child awakens during the night?	☐ yes ☐ no	**If yes,** do you think this is a problem?	☐ yes ☐ no

After nighttime awakening, child has difficulty falling back to sleep?	☐ yes ☐ no	**If yes**, do you think this is a problem?	☐ yes ☐ no
Child is difficult to awaken in the morning?	☐ yes ☐ no	**If yes**, do you think this is a problem?	☐ yes ☐ no
Child is a poor sleeper?	☐ yes ☐ no	**If yes**, do you think this is a problem?	☐ yes ☐ no

Current Sleep Symptoms						
						(f) do not know
					(e) always (6 to 7 nights/days a week)	
				(d) often (3 to 5 nights/days a week)		
			(c) sometimes (1 to 2 nights/days a week)			
		(b) not often (less than 1 night/day a week)				
		(a) never (does not happen)				
1.	Difficulty breathing when asleep	a	b	c	d	e	f
2.	Stops breathing during sleep	a	b	c	d	e	f
3.	Snores	a	b	c	d	e	f
4.	Restless sleep	a	b	c	d	e	f
5.	Sweating when sleeping	a	b	c	d	e	f
6.	Daytime sleepiness	a	b	c	d	e	f
7.	Poor appetite	a	b	c	d	e	f
8.	Nightmares	a	b	c	d	e	f
9.	Sleepwalking	a	b	c	d	e	f
10.	Sleeptalking	a	b	c	d	e	f
11.	Screaming in his/her sleep	a	b	c	d	e	f
12.	Kicks legs in sleep	a	b	c	d	e	f
13.	Wakes up at night	a	b	c	d	e	f
14.	Gets out of bed at night	a	b	c	d	e	f
15.	Trouble staying in his/her bed	a	b	c	d	e	f
16.	Resists going to bed at bedtime	a	b	c	d	e	f
17.	Grinds his/her teeth	a	b	c	d	e	f
18.	Uncomfortable feeling in his/her legs; creepy-crawly feeling	a	b	c	d	e	f
19.	Wets bed	a	b	c	d	e	f

Current Daytime Symptoms		(a) never (does not happen)	(b) not often (less than 1 day a week)	(c) sometimes (1 to 2 days a week)	(d) often (3 to 5 days a week)	(e) always (6 to 7 days a week)	(f) do not know
1.	Trouble getting up in the morning	a	b	c	d	e	f
2.	Falls asleep in school	a	b	c	d	e	f
3.	Naps after school	a	b	c	d	e	f
4.	Daytime sleepiness	a	b	c	d	e	f
5.	Feels weak or loses control of his/her muscles with strong emotions	a	b	c	d	e	f
6.	Reports unable to move when falling asleep or upon waking	a	b	c	d	e	f
7.	Sees frightening visual images before falling asleep or upon waking	a	b	c	d	e	f

PREGNANCY/ DELIVERY			
Pregnancy	☐ Normal	☐ Difficult	
Delivery	☐ Term	☐ Pre-term	☐ Post-term
Child's birthweight:			
Only child?	☐ Yes	☐ No If no, circle birth order: 1st 2nd 3rd 4th 5th 6th 7th	

MEDICAL AND PSYCHIATRIC HISTORY			
PAST MEDICAL HISTORY			
Frequent nasal congestion	☐ Yes	Age of diagnosis:	
Trouble breathing through his/her nose	☐ Yes	Age of diagnosis:	
Sinus problems	☐ Yes	Age of diagnosis:	
Chronic bronchitis or cough	☐ Yes	Age of diagnosis:	
Allergies	☐ Yes	Age of diagnosis:	Allergic to what:
Asthma	☐ Yes	Age of diagnosis:	
Frequent colds or flus	☐ Yes	Age of diagnosis:	
Frequent ear infections	☐ Yes	Age of diagnosis:	
Frequent strep throat infections	☐ Yes	Age of diagnosis:	
Difficulty swallowing	☐ Yes	Age of diagnosis:	
Acid reflux (gastroesophageal reflux)	☐ Yes	Age of diagnosis:	
Poor or delayed growth	☐ Yes	Age of diagnosis:	
Excessive weight	☐ Yes	Age of diagnosis:	
Hearing problems	☐ Yes	Age of diagnosis:	
Speech problems	☐ Yes	Age of diagnosis:	
Vision problems	☐ Yes	Age of diagnosis:	
Seizures/Epilepsy	☐ Yes	Age of diagnosis:	
Morning headaches	☐ Yes	Age of diagnosis:	
Cerebral palsy	☐ Yes	Age of diagnosis:	
Heart disease	☐ Yes	Age of diagnosis:	
High blood pressure	☐ Yes	Age of diagnosis:	
Sickle cell disease	☐ Yes	Age of diagnosis:	
Genetic disease	☐ Yes	Age of diagnosis:	
Chromosome problem (e.g., Down's)	☐ Yes	Age of diagnosis:	
Skeleton problem (e.g., dwarfism)	☐ Yes	Age of diagnosis:	
Cranofacial disorder (e.g., Pierre-Robin)	☐ Yes	Age of diagnosis:	
Thyroid problems	☐ Yes	Age of diagnosis:	
Eczema (itchy skin)	☐ Yes	Age of diagnosis:	
Pain	☐ Yes	Age of diagnosis:	

PAST PSYCHIATRIC/PSYCHOLOGICAL HISTORY

Autism	☐ Yes	Age of diagnosis:
Developmental delay	☐ Yes	Age of diagnosis:
Hyperactivity/ADHD	☐ Yes	Age of diagnosis:
Anxiety/Panic Attacks	☐ Yes	Age of diagnosis:
Obsessive Compulsive Disorder	☐ Yes	Age of diagnosis:
Depression	☐ Yes	Age of diagnosis:
Suicide	☐ Yes	Age of diagnosis:
Learning disability	☐ Yes	Age of diagnosis:
Drug use/abuse	☐ Yes	Age of diagnosis:
Behavioral disorder	☐ Yes	Age of diagnosis:
Psychiatric Admission	☐ Yes	Age of diagnosis:

Please list any additional psychological, psychiatric, emotional, or behavioral problems diagnosed or suspected by a physician/psychologist.

CURRENT MEDICAL HISTORY

Please list any medications your child currently takes:

Medicine	Dose	How often?
1.		
2.		
3.		
4.		

LONG-TERM MEDICAL PROBLEMS

If your child has long-term medical problems, please list the three you think are most important.

1.

2.

3.

SURGERIES/HOSPITALIZATIONS

Has your child ever had his/her tonsils removed?	☐ Yes	Age of surgery:
Has your child ever had his/her adenoids removed?	☐ Yes	Age of surgery:
Has your child ever had ear tubes?	☐ Yes	Age of surgery:

Please list any additional hospitalizations or surgeries:

HEALTH HABITS

Does your child drink caffeinated beverages? (e.g., Coke, Pepsi, Mountain Dew, iced tea)	☐ No	☐ Yes	Amount per day:

SCHOOL PERFORMANCE

CURRENT SCHOOL PERFORMANCE (if school-aged)

Your child's grade:					
Has your child ever repeated a grade?	☐ No	☐ Yes			
Is your child enrolled in any special education class?	☐ No	☐ Yes			
How many school days has your child missed so far this year?					
How many school days did your child miss last year?					
How many school days was your child late so far this year?					
How many school days was your child late last year?					
Child's grades this year:	☐ Excellent	☐ Good	☐ Average	☐ Poor	☐ Failing
Child's grades last year:	☐ Excellent	☐ Good	☐ Average	☐ Poor	☐ Failing

FAMILY'S INFORMATION	
MOTHER	**FATHER**
Age:	Age:
Marital Status: ☐ Single ☐ Divorced ☐ Separated ☐ Married ☐ Widowed ☐ Remarried	Marital Status: ☐ Single ☐ Divorced ☐ Separated ☐ Married ☐ Widowed ☐ Remarried
Education:	Education:
Work: ☐ Unemployed ☐ Part-time ☐ Full-time	Work: ☐ Unemployed ☐ Part-time ☐ Full-time
Occupation:	Occupation:

PERSONS LIVING IN HOME

Name:	Relationship	Age

FAMILY SLEEP HISTORY

Does anyone in the family have a sleep disorder?   ☐ Yes   ☐ No

If yes, mark the disorder(s):

Insomnia	☐ Mother	☐ Father	☐ Brother/sister	☐ Grandparent
Snoring	☐ Mother	☐ Father	☐ Brother/sister	☐ Grandparent
Sleep apnea	☐ Mother	☐ Father	☐ Brother/sister	☐ Grandparent
Restless legs syndrome	☐ Mother	☐ Father	☐ Brother/sister	☐ Grandparent
Periodic limb movement disorder	☐ Mother	☐ Father	☐ Brother/sister	☐ Grandparent
Sleepwalking/sleep terrors	☐ Mother	☐ Father	☐ Brother/sister	☐ Grandparent
Sleep talking	☐ Mother	☐ Father	☐ Brother/sister	☐ Grandparent
Narcolepsy	☐ Mother	☐ Father	☐ Brother/sister	☐ Grandparent
Other:	☐ Mother	☐ Father	☐ Brother/sister	☐ Grandparent

REFERRAL

Who asked that your child be seen by a sleep specialist?

_____ Pediatrician/Family physician

_____ Child's parent or guardian

_____ Surgical specialist (e.g., ENT)

_____ Pediatric specialist (e.g., allergist, neurologist, pulmonolgist)

_____ Mental health specialist (e.g. psychiatrist, psychologist, social worker)

_____ School teacher, nurse, counselor

_____ Child himself/herself

_____ Other:

Appendix B

Sleep Diaries

PEDIATRIC SLEEP LOG

Your name: _____

Your birth date: ___ / ___ / ___

↓ Mark your bedtime and any nap times with downward arrows. →

Shade in the periods when you were asleep

Example:

Date	Day																			
	1																			
	2																			

↑ Mark the time you get up in the morning and after any naps with upward arrrows.

Date	Day	Mid night		2 AM		4 AM		6 AM		8 AM		10 AM		Noon		2 PM		4 PM		6 PM		8 PM		10 PM		Mid Night

Sleep Diary

Every morning when you get up complete the sleep diary for the previous night. For example, on Monday morning fill in the information for Sunday night.

Day	Last night I went to bed at:	This morning I woke up at:	It took me ___ minutes to fall asleep:	Total amount of sleep:
Example: Sunday	12:15	9:20	25	9' 10"

DAY: _____

Morning

Time child woke in AM: _____
Time child got out of bed: _____

Child was woken by: Self
                     Parent
                     Sibling/other
                     Alarm

Mood on waking: 1 2 3 4 5 **(circle one)**

    Unhappy   **Happy**

Naps and Daytime Sleepiness

Time(s) and lengths of planned nap(s) during the day: _____

Did child fall asleep today (check all that apply):

_____ riding in the car?
_____ watching TV?
_____ while eating?
_____ while playing?
_____ in school?
_____ other? Please describe _____

Bedtime

Time went to bed in PM ("lights out"): _____

Describe any problems going to bed: _____
_____
_____
_____

Time child actually fell asleep: _____

Night Wakings

Time(s) and length(s) of night wakings:
Time awoke: 1) _____   Back to sleep: 1) _____   Brief describe what happened:1) _____
         2)   2)   2)
         3)   3)   3)
         4)   4)   4)

Appendix C

Screening Questionnaire for Obstructive Sleep Apnea

Screening Questionnaire: Obstructive Sleep Apnea

Name: _____
Person completing form: _____   Date: ___/___/___

Please answer the following questions as they pertain to your child in the past month.

1. **While sleeping, does your child:**

    Snore more than half the time?.. Y   N   DK

    Always snore?   ....Y   N   DK

    Snore loudly?   ....Y   N   DK

    Have "heavy" or loud breathing? ....Y   N   DK

    Have trouble breathing, or struggle to breathe? ....Y   N   DK

2. **Have you ever seen your child stop breathing during
    the night?** .... Y   N   DK

3. **Does your child:**

    Tend to breathe through the mouth during the day?.................Y   N   DK

    Have a dry mouth on waking up in the morning? ....Y   N   DK

    Occasionally wet the bed? ....Y   N   DK

4. **Does your child:**

    Wake up feeling unrefreshed in the morning? ....Y   N   DK

    Have a problem with sleepiness during the day? ....Y   N   DK

5. **Has a teacher or other supervisor commented that your
    child appears sleepy during the day?** ....Y   N DK

6. **Is it hard to wake your child up in the morning?** ....Y   N   DK

7. **Does your child wake up with headaches in the morning?** ....Y   N DK

8. **Did your child stop growing at a normal rate at
    any time since birth?** ....   Y   N   DK

9. **Is your child overweight?** ....   Y   N   DK

10. **This child *often*:**

Does not seem to listen when spoken to directly. ……………………………...Y   N   DK

Has difficulty organizing tasks and activities. …………………………….……..Y   N   DK

Is easily distracted by extraneous stimuli. ……………………………….……..Y   N   DK

Fidgets with hands or feet or squirms in seat. …………………………….....Y   N   DK

Is "on the go" or often acts as if "driven by a motor". …………………….…Y   N   DK

Interrupts or intrudes on others (eg., butts into conversations or games). ………Y   N   DK

Scoring

Yes = 1
No = 0

Average all scores to obtain a score between 0.00 and 1.00. Preliminary analyses suggest a cut-off of >0.33 for abnormal.

(For more information see Chervin RD, Hedger K, Dillon JE, Pituch KJ (2000). Pediatric Sleep Questionnaire (PSQ): validity and reliability of scales for sleep-disordered breathing, snoring, sleepiness, and behavioral problems. Sleep Medicine1:21-32.)

Appendix D

Screening Questionnaire for Restless Legs Syndrome

Screening Questionnaire:

Restless Legs Syndrome
(Parent Version)

Child's Name _____

Person filling out form (circle one):   Mother   Father   Other (specify): _____

1. Does your child have "growing pains"? (Check One)

_____ never _____ occasionally _____ sometimes _____ frequently
(less than 1x/month   (1-2x/month)   (1-2x/wk to daily)

2. Does your child complain of uncomfortable or funny feelings (creeping, crawling, tingling) in his/her legs? (Check One)

_____ never _____ occasionally _____ sometimes _____ frequently
(less than 1x/month   (1-2x/month)   (1-2x/wk to daily)

	YES	NO	DON'T KNOW
3. Does your child:			
A. Notice funny feelings in his/her legs (or do they seem worse) when lying down or sitting?	____	____	____
B. Have partial relief with movement (wiggling feet, toes, or walking?)	____	____	____
C. Complain that the feelings are worse at night?	____	____	____
D. Have a lot of fidgeting or wiggling of the feet or toes when sitting or lying down?	____	____	____
E. Have repeated jerking movements in toes or legs or the whole body while sleeping?	____	____	____

4. Does your child appear restless while sleeping (thrashing around, banging feet against wall. twisting covers, or falling out of bed)? (Check One)

_____ never _____ occasionally _____ sometimes _____ frequently
(less than 1x/month (1-2x/month) (1-2x/wk to daily)

5. Does your child seem more restless, fidgety or hyperactive than most children his/her age?

_____ never _____ occasionally _____ sometimes _____ frequently
(less than 1x/month (1-2x/month) (1-2x/wk to daily)

6a. Has anyone in the family (including grandparents, aunts/uncles) been diagnosed with restless legs or periodic leg movements during sleep? _____Yes _____No

If so, who: _____

6b. Does anyone in the family have severe problems falling or staying asleep? If so, who:
_____. Type of problem, if known: _____

7. How often, on average, does your child consume caffeine-containing beverages or food? (coffee, tea, cola beverages, chocolate)

_____ never _____ occasionally _____ sometimes _____ frequently
(less than 1x/month (1-2x/month) (1-2x/wk to daily)

8. Has your child ever been diagnosed and/or treated for anemia? Yes___ No___ Don't Know___
Date, type of anemia, and treatment, if known:_____

Restless Legs Syndrome
(Adolescent Self-Report Version)

Your name:

_____

1. Have you ever had "growing pains"? (Check one)

   ____ never ____ occasionally ____ sometimes ____ frequently ____ only in the past
              (less than 1x/month)   (1-2x/month)   (1-2x/wk to daily)

2. Do you have uncomfortable or funny feelings (creeping, crawling, tingling) in your legs? (Check one)

   ____ never ____ occasionally ____ sometimes ____ frequently ____ only in the past
              (less than 1x/month)   (1-2x/month)   (1-2x/wk to daily)

3. Do you ever:

	YES	NO	DON'T KNOW
A. Notice funny feelings in your legs (or do they seem worse) when lying down or sitting?	☐	☐	☐
B. Have partial relief with movement (wiggling feet, toes, or walking?)	☐	☐	☐
C. Notice that the feeling is worse at night?	☐	☐	☐
D. Have a lot of fidgeting or wiggling of your feet or toes when sitting or lying down?	☐	☐	☐
E. Have repeated jerking movements in toes or legs or the whole body while sleeping?	☐	☐	☐

Appendix E

General Sleep Handouts

Appendix E1

Sleep in Newborns
(0–2 Months)

WHAT TO EXPECT

Newborns sleep between 11 and 18 hours per day, with no regular or defined pattern. For the first few weeks, your baby will sleep for anywhere from a few minutes to a few hours at a time, although babies who are breast-fed tend to sleep for shorter periods (2–3 hours of sleep) than bottle-fed babies (3–4 hours). There will also be little difference between night and day in the first few weeks. However, you will start to see a more regular sleep schedule develop between 2 and 4 months of age. Expect your baby to be quite active while she sleeps. All babies smile, grimace, suck, snuffle, and move (twitch, jerk) while they sleep. This is perfectly normal, and your baby is getting sound sleep.

WHERE AND HOW SHOULD YOUR BABY SLEEP?

- **Sleeping arrangements.** There are many choices as to where your newborn sleeps, whether in a bassinet or a crib in the parents' bedroom, a sibling's bedroom, or the baby's own room. Some parents prefer to have their baby sleep with them, although caution should be taken as there is a risk of suffocation.
- **Back to sleep.** All babies should be put to sleep on their backs to reduce the risk of sudden infant death syndrome (SIDS).

Safe Sleep Practices for Newborns

- Place your baby on his or her back to sleep at night and during naptime.
- Place your baby on a firm mattress in a safety-approved crib with slats no greater than 2-⅜ inches apart.
- Make sure your baby's face and head stay uncovered and clear of blankets and other coverings during sleep. If a blanket is used, make sure your baby is placed "feet-to-foot" (feet at the bottom of the crib, blanket no higher than chest-level, blanket tucked in around mattress) in the crib. Remove all pillows from the crib.
- Create a "smoke-free–zone" around your baby.
- Avoid overheating during sleep and maintain your baby's bedroom at a temperature comfortable for an average adult.

HOW TO HELP YOUR NEWBORN BECOME A GOOD SLEEPER

- **Learn your baby's signs of being sleepy.** Some babies fuss or cry when they are tired, whereas others rub their eyes, stare off into space, or pull on their ears. Your baby will fall asleep more easily and more quickly if you put him down to sleep when he lets you know that he is tired.
- **Encourage nighttime sleep.** Many newborns have their days and nights reversed, sleeping much of the day and being awake much of the night. To help your baby sleep more at night, keep lights dim during the night and keep play to a minimum. During the day, play with your baby and be sure to wake him regularly for feedings and play time.
- **Respond to your baby's sleep needs.** Newborns often need to be rocked or fed to sleep, which is fine for the first few weeks or months. However, once your baby is 3 months old, begin to establish good sleep habits.
- **Develop a bedtime routine.** Even babies as young as a few weeks respond well to bedtime routines. Your newborn's bedtime routine should be soothing and can include any activities you choose, such as bathing, rocking, and cuddling.
- **Sleep when your baby sleeps.** Parents need sleep also. Try to nap when your baby naps, and be sure to ask others for help so that you can get some rest.
- **Contact your doctor if you are concerned.** Babies who are extremely fussy or frequently difficult to console may have a medical problem, such as colic or reflux. Also, be sure to contact your doctor if your baby ever seems to have problems breathing.

Appendix E2

Sleep in Infants
(2–12 Months)

WHAT TO EXPECT

Infants sleep between 9 and 12 hours during the night and nap between 2 and 5 hours during the day. At 2 months, infants take between two and four naps each day, and by 12 months, they take either one or two naps. Expect factors such as illness or a change in routine to disrupt your baby's sleep. Developmental milestones, including pulling to standing and crawling, may also temporarily disrupt sleep.

By 6 months of age, most babies are physiologically capable of sleeping through the night and no longer require nighttime feedings. However, 25%–50% continue to awaken during the night. When it comes to waking during the night, the most important point to understand is that all babies wake briefly between four and six times. Babies who are able to soothe themselves back to sleep ("self-soothers") awaken briefly and go right back to sleep. In contrast, "signalers" are those babies who awaken their parents and need help getting back to sleep. Many of these signalers have developed inappropriate sleep onset associations and thus have difficulty self-soothing. This is often the result of parents developing the habit of helping their baby to fall asleep by rocking, holding, or bringing the child into their own bed. Over time, babies may learn to rely on this kind of help from their parents in order to fall asleep. Although this may not be a problem at bedtime, it may lead to difficulties with your baby failing back to sleep on her own during the night.

Safe Sleep Practices for Infants

- Place your baby on his or her back to sleep at night and during naptime.
- Place your baby on a firm mattress in a safety-approved crib with slats no greater than 2-⅜ inches apart.
- Make sure your baby's face and head stay uncovered and clear of blankets and other coverings during sleep. If a blanket is used, make sure the baby is placed "feet-to-foot" (feet at the bottom of the crib, blanket no higher than chest-level, blanket tucked in around mattress) in the crib. Remove all pillows from the crib.
- Create a "smoke-free–zone" around your baby.
- Avoid overheating during sleep and maintain your baby's bedroom at a temperature comfortable for an average adult.
- Remove all mobiles and hanging crib toys by about the age of 5 months, when your baby begins to pull up in the crib.
- Remove crib bumpers by about 12 months, when your baby can begin to climb.

HOW TO HELP YOUR INFANT SLEEP WELL

- **Learn your baby's signs of being sleepy.** Some babies fuss or cry when they are tired, whereas others rub their eyes, stare off into space, or pull on their ears. Your baby will fall asleep more easily and more quickly if you put her down the minute she lets you know that she is sleepy.
- **Decide on where your baby is going to sleep.** Try to decide where your baby is going to sleep for the long run by 3 months of age, as changes in sleeping arrangements will be harder on your baby as he gets older. For example, if your baby is sleeping in a bassinet, move him to a crib by 3 months. If your baby is sharing your bed, decide whether to continue that arrangement.
- **Develop a daily sleep schedule.** Babies sleep best when they have consistent sleep times and wake times. Note that cutting back on naps to encourage nighttime sleep results in overtiredness and a worse night's sleep.
- **Encourage use of a security object.** Once your baby is old enough (by 12 months), introduce a transitional/love object, such as a stuffed animal, a blanket, or a t-shirt that was worn by you (tie it in a knot). Include it as part of your bedtime routine and whenever you are cuddling or comforting your baby. Don't force your baby to accept the object, and realize that some babies never develop an attachment to a single item.
- **Develop a bedtime routine.** Establish a consistent bedtime routine that includes calm and enjoyable activities, such as a bath and bedtime stories, and that you can stick with as your baby gets older. The activities occurring clos-

est to "lights out" should occur in the room where your baby sleeps. Also, avoid making bedtime feedings part of the bedtime routine after 6 months.

- **Set up a consistent bedroom environment.** Make sure your child's bedroom environment is the same at bedtime as it is throughout the night (e.g., lighting). Also, babies sleep best in a room that is dark, cool, and quiet.
- **Put your baby to bed drowsy but awake.** After your bedtime routine, put your baby to bed drowsy but awake, which will encourage her to fall asleep independently. This will teach your baby to soothe herself to sleep, so that she will be able to fall back to sleep on her own when she naturally awakens during the night.
- **Sleep when your baby sleeps.** Parents need sleep also. Try to nap when your baby naps, and be sure to ask others for help so you can get some rest.
- **Contact your doctor if you are concerned.** Babies who are extremely fussy or frequently difficult to console may have a medical problem, such as colic or reflux. Also, be sure to contact your doctor if your baby ever seems to have problems breathing.

Appendix E3

Sleep in Toddlers (1–3 Years)

WHAT TO EXPECT

Toddlers sleep between 12 and 14 hours across the day and night. By 18 months, most toddlers have given up their morning nap and are taking one long afternoon nap of 1.5–3 hours. The number of hours a toddler sleeps will be different for each child, but expect your toddler to sleep about the same amount each day. Continue to expect that sleep will be disrupted by illness, changes in routine, and other stressful events. Separation anxiety may also cause problems at bedtime. Most toddlers switch from a crib to a bed between 2 and 3 years of age. If the change happens too early, it can disrupt sleep.

Many toddlers continue to awaken during the night, usually as a result of poor sleep habits. All children wake briefly throughout the night. However, a toddler who has not learned how to fall asleep on his own at bedtime will not be able to return to sleep without help from his parents.

HOW TO HELP YOUR TODDLER SLEEP WELL

- **Develop a daily sleep schedule.** Have regular nap times and a bedtime that ensures enough nighttime sleep. Napping too late in the afternoon can make it hard for your toddler to fall asleep at bedtime, but avoid cutting back on naps to encourage nighttime sleep as this will result in overtiredness and a worse night's sleep.
- **Encourage use of a security object.** Helping your toddler become attached to a security object that he can keep in bed with him can be beneficial. This often helps a child feel more relaxed at bedtime and throughout the night.
- **Develop a bedtime routine.** Establish a consistent bedtime routine that includes calm and enjoyable activities, such as a bath and bedtime stories. The activities occurring closest to "lights out" should occur in the room where your toddler sleeps.

- **Set up a consistent bedroom environment.** Make sure your child's bedroom environment is the same at bedtime as it is throughout the night. Some older toddlers may find a nightlight reassuring. Also, toddlers sleep best in a room that is dark, cool, and quiet.
- **Put your toddler to bed drowsy but awake.** Encourage your toddler to fall asleep independently by putting him to bed drowsy but awake. This will enable him to fall back to sleep on his own when he naturally awakens during the night.
- **Set limits.** If your toddler stalls at bedtime, be sure to set clear limits, such as how many books you will read.
- **Contact your child's doctor if:**
  - Your child appears to have any trouble breathing, snores, or is a noisy breather.
  - Your child has unusual nighttime awakenings or significant nighttime fears that are concerning.
  - Your child has difficulty falling asleep, staying asleep, and/or if sleep problems are affecting his behavior during the day.

Appendix E4

Sleep in Preschoolers (3–5 Years)

WHAT TO EXPECT:

Preschoolers need between 11 and 13 hours of sleep. The number of hours a preschooler sleeps will be different for each child, but expect your preschooler to sleep for about the same amount of time each day. Most preschoolers stop taking naps between 3 and 5 years of age. Some preschoolers continue to awaken during the night, usually as a result of poor sleep habits. All children wake briefly throughout the night. However, a preschooler who has not learned how to fall asleep on her own at bedtime will not be able to return to sleep without help from her parents.

Sleep problems are common during the preschool years, including nighttime fears and nightmares. Nighttime fears and nightmares are a part of normal development. Sleepwalking and sleep terrors are also common during the preschool years and peak in this age group.

HOW TO HELP YOUR PRESCHOOLER SLEEP WELL

- **Develop a regular sleep schedule.** Your preschooler should go to bed and wake up about the same time each day. You may find that your preschooler has a "second wind" in the evening. Move bedtime earlier or later to a time when your child is more physiologically ready for sleep. Also, be sure that your child is ready for sleep before putting her to bed. This may seem obvious, but sometimes parents set a bedtime based on their own convenience. For example, some children's biological clocks make them more likely to be "night owls." These children may have difficulty with an earlier bedtime.
- **Maintain a consistent bedtime routine.** Establish a bedtime routine that is the same every night and includes calm and enjoyable activities, such as a bath and bedtime stories. The activities occurring closest to "lights out" should occur in the room where your preschooler sleeps.

- **Set up a soothing sleep environment.** Make sure your child's bedroom is comfortable, dark, cool, and quiet. A nightlight is fine; a television is not.
- **Set limits.** If your preschooler stalls at bedtime, be sure to set clear limits, such as how many books you will read.
- **Contact your child's doctor if:**
  - Your child appears to have any trouble breathing, snores, or is a noisy breather.
  - Your child has unusual nighttime awakenings or significant nighttime fears that are concerning.
  - Your child has difficulty falling asleep, staying asleep, and/or if her sleep problems are affecting her behavior during the day.

Appendix E5

Sleep in School-Aged Children (6–12 Years)

WHAT TO EXPECT

School-aged children need between 10 and 11 hours of sleep per night. Not getting enough sleep is common in this age group, given increasing school obligations (e.g., homework), evening activities, and later bedtimes. Sleep problems are also common in the school-aged child, including sleepwalking, sleep terrors, teeth grinding, nighttime fears, snoring, and noisy breathing.

Signs of sleep deprivation in school-aged children can include:

- **Mood.** Sleep deprivation may cause your school-aged child to be moody, irritable, and cranky. In addition, he may have a difficult time regulating his mood, such as by getting frustrated or upset more easily.
- **Behavior.** School-aged children who do not get enough sleep are more likely to have behavior problems, such as noncompliance and hyperactivity.
- **Cognitive ability.** Inadequate sleep may result in problems with attention, memory, decision making, reaction time, and creativity, all which are important in school.

HOW TO HELP YOUR SCHOOL-AGED CHILD SLEEP WELL

- **Develop a regular sleep schedule.** Your child should go to bed and wake up at about the same time each day.
- **Maintain a consistent bedtime routine.** School-aged children continue to benefit from a bedtime routine that is the same every night and includes calm and enjoyable activities. Including one-on-one time with a parent is helpful in maintaining communication with your child and having a clear connection every day.
- **Set up a soothing sleep environment.** Make sure your child's bedroom is comfortable, dark, cool, and quiet. A nightlight is fine; a television is not.

- **Set limits.** If your school-aged child stalls at bedtime, be sure to set clear limits, such as what time lights must be turned off and how many bedtime stories you will read.
- **Turn off televisions, computers, and radios.** Television viewing, computer-game playing, internet use, and other stimulating activities at bedtime will cause sleep problems.
- **Avoid caffeine.** Caffeine can be found in sodas, coffee-based products, iced tea, and many other substances.
- **Contact your child's doctor.** Speak to your child's physician if your child has difficulties falling asleep or staying asleep, snores, experiences unusual awakenings, or has sleep problems that are causing disruption during the day.

Appendix E6

Sleep in Adolescents (13–18 Years)

WHAT TO EXPECT

Adolescents are notorious for not getting enough sleep. The average amount of sleep that teenagers get is between 7 and 7¼ hours. However, they need between 9 and 9½ hours (studies show that most teenagers need exactly 9¼ hours of sleep). Teenagers do not get enough sleep for a number of reasons:

- **Shift in sleep schedule.** After puberty, there is a biological shift in an adolescent's internal clock of about 2 hours, meaning that a teenager who used to fall asleep at 9:00 PM will now not be able to fall asleep until 11:00 PM. It also means waking 2 hours later in the morning.
- **Early high school start times.** In most school districts, the move to high school is accompanied by an earlier school start time. Some high schools start as early as 7:00 AM, meaning that some teenagers have to get up as early as 5:00 AM to get ready for and travel to school.
- **Social and school obligations.** Homework, sports, after-school activities (often occurring during the evening), and socializing lead to late bedtimes.

As a result, most adolescents are very sleep deprived. Sleep deprivation will impact on many aspects of your teenager's functioning:

- **Mood.** Sleep deprivation will cause your teenager to be moody, irritable, and cranky. In addition, she will have a difficult time regulating her mood, such as getting frustrated or upset more easily.
- **Behavior.** Teenagers who are sleep deprived are also more likely to engage in risk-taking behaviors, such as drinking, driving fast, and engaging in other dangerous activities.
- **Cognitive ability.** Inadequate sleep will result in problems with attention, memory, decision making, reaction time, and creativity, all of which are important in school.

- **Academic performance.** Studies show that teenagers who get less sleep are more apt to get poor grades in school, fall asleep in school, and have school tardiness/absences.
- **Drowsy driving.** Teenagers are at the highest risk for falling asleep at the wheel. Drowsy driving is most likely to occur in the middle of the night (2:00 to 4:00 AM), but also in mid-afternoon (3:00 to 4:00 PM).

HOW TO HELP YOUR TEENAGER GET ENOUGH SLEEP

- **Maintain a regular sleep schedule.** Your teenager should go to bed and wake up at about the same time each day. Her sleep schedule should also ensure adequate time in bed.
- **Avoid oversleeping on weekends.** Although catching up on some sleep on the weekends can be helpful, sleeping in until noon on Sunday will make it hard for your teenager to get back on a school schedule that night.
- **Take early afternoon naps.** A nap of 30–45 minutes in the early afternoon can be beneficial.
- **Turn off televisions, computers, and radios.** Television viewing, computer-game playing, internet use, and other stimulating activities at bedtime will cause problems falling asleep.
- **Avoid caffeine, smoking, alcohol, and drugs.** All of these cause sleep problems.
- **Contact your teenager's doctor.** Speak to your adolescent's physician if she has difficulties falling asleep or staying asleep, snores, or seems excessively sleepy during the day.

Appendix F

Sleep Disorders Handouts

Appendix F1

Bedtime Problems

Getting a child to go to bed is a common problem that many parents experience. Some children use stalling and excuses to resist going to bed, whereas others go to bed initially but do not stay there. Bedtime problems can be one of the most frustrating parts of a parent's day. Bedtime problems can occur at any age but are most prevalent between 3 and 6 years.

WHAT CAN YOU DO TO HELP YOUR CHILD GO TO BED?

First of all, it is important to realize that you cannot "make" a child go to sleep. However, you can help your child improve his bedtime behavior and help him to get to sleep more easily and quickly. As with many other skills your child needs to learn, this will take time.

- **Stick to firm bedtime limits.** The first step is to be convinced that your child needs to change his bedtime behavior, and that setting and sticking to firm bedtime limits is in everyone's best interest, especially your child's. Setting limits is an important part of parenting. Children do not have a lot of self-control yet, and so they benefit from the structure of limits that you set for them. This helps them to learn self-control. In addition, limits relieve (not cause) anxiety in children. Finally, prepare yourself for some hard work. Changing behavior is always difficult. Your child is probably happy with bedtime the way it is and so will initially have little motivation to change. You need to be consistent and persistent.
- **Explain the new rules to your child.** Before you start the new nighttime program, sit down with your child during the day and let him know what you expect. Do not make your conversation too long or involved and do not over-explain. Ignore any negative comments by your child and avoid arguing about the new rules.
- **Set bedtime.** Once you have decided on your child's bedtime, be *consistent* about it. Establish a regular bedtime to help set your child's internal clock. Be sure that your child is ready for sleep before putting him to bed. This may seem obvious, but sometimes parents set a bedtime for their own convenience.

For example, some children's biological clocks make them more likely to be "night owls." These children may have difficulty with an earlier bedtime.

- **Bedtime fading.** Putting children to bed when they are not tired increases the likelihood of bedtime struggles. Therefore, for some children, it is best to start by setting the bedtime at the time they usually fall asleep and gradually make the bedtime earlier. When you start, you will first need to determine when your child is naturally falling asleep and set this as his *temporary* bedtime. If you would like your child to go to bed at 8:30, but he usually does not fall asleep until 10:30, choose 10:30 as his temporary bedtime. This will make it easier to teach your child how to fall asleep within a short time of getting into bed. Once he is falling asleep easily and quickly at his temporary bedtime, then you can start making his bedtime earlier by 15 minutes every few days. Be patient. If you move the bedtime back too quickly, you may have problems with your child not being able to fall asleep.
- **Bedtime routine.** Be sure to establish a consistent bedtime routine. A bedtime routine should include calm and enjoyable activities, such as a bath and bedtime stories. Avoid stimulating high-energy activities, such as playing outside, running around, or watching exciting television shows or videos. Make a chart of your bedtime routine to help keep your child on track. Also, having the last part of the bedtime routine be a favorite activity will help motivate your child to get ready for bed.
- **Ignore complaints or protests.** Ignore your child's complaints or protests about bedtime, such as not being tired. Discussing or arguing about bedtime will lead to a struggle with your child, thus maintaining bedtime problems. Firmly and calmly let your child know it is time for bed and continue with the routine.
- **Putting your child to bed.** When the bedtime routine is complete, put your child to bed and leave the room. It is important that you leave the room while your child is awake, as this helps your child learn to fall asleep on his own.
- **If your child cries or yells.** If your child is yelling or calling out to you but remaining in his bed, remind him one time that it is bedtime. If he continues to be upset, check on your child. Wait for as long or short a time as you wish. For some children, checking frequently is effective; for others, checking infrequently works best. Continue returning to check on your child as long as he is crying or upset. The visits should be *brief* (1 minute) and *boring*. Don't soothe or comfort your child during these visits and don't get into a discussion. Calmly tell your child that it's time to go to sleep. The purpose of returning to the room is to reassure your child that you are still present and to reassure you that your child is okay.
- **What to do if your child gets out of bed or comes out of his room.** If your child gets out of bed or comes out of his room, firmly and calmly return him to bed. For some children, simply returning them to bed multiple times works. For others, letting him know that if he gets up again, you will close the bedroom door can be effective. If your child gets out of bed, put him back in bed

and close the door for a brief period (1 minute to start). After the allotted time, open the door. If your child is in bed, praise him and leave the door open. If he is up, put him back in bed and close the door again but leave it closed for a longer time, increasing the time by a few minutes each time he gets up.

- **Don't lock your child in his room.** Locking the door may be scary for your child. The goal is to teach your child to stay in bed, not punish or scare him.
- **Reward your child.** Soon after your child awakens in the morning, reward him for what he did well the night before. Don't dwell on misbehavior from the previous night. Give your attention to your child's successes. Stickers, praise, and breakfast treats are good ways to reward your child for even small improvements.
- **Be consistent and don't give up.** The first few nights are likely to be very challenging. You should start to see major improvements within the first few weeks.

Appendix F2

Nightwakings

Nightwakings in young children is one of the most common problems that parents face. By 6 months of age, most babies are physiologically capable of sleeping throughout the night and no longer require nighttime feedings. However, 25%–50% continue to awaken during the night. Nightwaking problems can occur at any age but are most common with infants and toddlers.

WHY DOES YOUR CHILD WAKE DURING THE NIGHT?

When it comes to nightwaking, the most important thing for parents to understand is that all children, no matter the age, wake briefly throughout the night. These arousals occur between four to six times per night. So the problem is rarely the waking during the night but rather why the child is unable to return to sleep on her own. Children who are able to soothe themselves back to sleep ("self-soothers") awaken briefly throughout the night, but their parents are unaware of these arousals. In contrast, "signalers" are those children who alert their parents by crying or going into the parents' bedroom upon awakening. Many of these "signaler" children have developed inappropriate sleep-onset associations and, thus, have difficulty self-soothing.

WHAT ARE SLEEP ASSOCIATIONS?

Many parents develop the habit of helping their child to fall asleep by rocking, holding, or bringing the child into bed with them. Over time, children may learn to rely on this kind of help from their parents in order to fall asleep. Although this may not be a problem at bedtime, it may lead to difficulties with your child failing back to sleep on her own during the night. Thus, sleep associations are conditions that the child *learns to need* in order to fall asleep at bedtime (such as rocking, nursing, or lying next to a parent). These same sleep associations are then needed in order to *fall back to sleep* during the night. The bottom line is that your child needs to learn to fall asleep on her own, so that she can put herself immediately back to sleep when she awakens.

WHAT CAN YOU DO TO HELP YOUR CHILD SLEEP THROUGH THE NIGHT?

There are a number of steps that you can take to help your child sleep through the night:

- **Develop an appropriate sleep schedule with an early bedtime.** Ironically, the more tired your child is, the more times she will awaken during the night. So be sure to have your child continue to take naps during the day and set an early bedtime.
- **Security object.** Try to introduce your child to a transitional/love object. A transitional object, like a stuffed toy, doll, or blanket, helps a child feel safe and secure when you are not present. Help your child become attached to a transitional object by including it as part of the bedtime routine. Try to include this object whenever you are cuddling or comforting your child. Don't force your child to accept the object, and realize that some children will not accept one no matter how cute and cuddly the object.
- **Bedtime routine.** Establish a consistent bedtime routine that includes calm and enjoyable activities, such as a bath and bedtime stories. Avoid exciting high-energy activities, such as playing outside, running around, or watching television shows or videos. The activities occurring closest to "lights out" should occur in the room where your child sleeps. Also, avoid making bedtime feedings part of the bedtime routine after 6 months.
- **Consistent bedroom environment.** Make sure your child's bedroom environment is the same at bedtime as it is throughout the night (e.g., lighting).
- **Put your child to bed drowsy but awake.** After the bedtime routine, put your child in her crib/bed drowsy but awake and leave the room. Remember, the key to having your child sleep through the night is to have her learn to fall asleep on her own, so she can put herself back to sleep when she naturally awakens during the night.
- **Checking method.** If your child cries or yells, check on her. Wait for as long or as short a time as you wish. For some children, frequent checking is effective; for others, infrequent checking works best. Continue returning to check on your child as long as she is crying or upset. The visits should be *brief* (1 minute) and *boring*. Calmly tell your child it's time to go to sleep. The purpose of returning to the room is to reassure your child that you are still present and to reassure you that your child is okay.
- **Respond to your child during the night.** In the beginning, respond to your child as you normally do throughout the night (e.g., nurse, rock). Research indicates that the majority of children will naturally begin sleeping through the night within 1–2 weeks of falling asleep quickly and easily at bedtime. If your child continues to awaken during the night after several weeks, then use the same checking method during the night as you did at bedtime.
- **A more gradual approach.** Some parents feel that not being present when their baby falls asleep feels like too big of a first step for them and their baby.

A more gradual approach is to teach your baby to fall asleep on her own but with you in the room. This approach will take longer but feels more comfortable to some families. The first step is to put your child in her crib/bed awake and sit on a chair next to the crib/bed. Once she is able to consistently fall asleep this way, sit farther and farther away every three to four nights until you are finally in the hallway and no longer in sight.

- **Be consistent and don't give up.** The first few nights are likely to be very challenging and often the second or third night is worse than the first night. However, within a few nights to a week, you will begin to see improvement.

Appendix F3

Nighttime Fears

It is normal for children to have nighttime fears, especially at bedtime, and most children have these at some point. Bedtime fears are normal and part of normal development. Fear of the dark, and other nighttime fears, develop as children begin to understand that they can get hurt or be harmed. Children have different fears at different developmental stages; for example, many young children are afraid of monsters. In addition, younger children, in particular, cannot always distinguish what is real from what is imagined.

WHAT TO DO WHEN YOUR CHILD IS AFRAID AT BEDTIME (OR OTHER TIMES OF THE NIGHT)

Dealing with a child who is afraid of the dark or scared to go to bed at night can be like walking a tightrope. There is a fine line between wanting to reassure him and not wanting to reinforce his fears. If the fears are ignored, the child will not be reassured. If the child is reassured too much, the parent may be giving the subtle message that there is something to fear. If bedtime fears are affecting your child's ability to fall asleep and stay asleep, try some of the following:

- **Listen and understand.** Try to understand your child's fears. Don't dismiss or make fun of them because fears that seem silly to an adult may be very real to a child.
- **Reassure your child.** It is important to reassure children who are fearful. When your child clings to you as he is being tucked in or calls out in fear, you should go back to his bed and find out what is wrong. Say something like, "You are safe; we are here to make sure you stay safe." Be sure to communicate that he is safe over and over again.
- **Teach coping skills.** Teach your child coping skills and discuss alternative ways to respond to nighttime fears, such as by "being brave" and thinking positive thoughts (e.g., "monsters are just pretend"). You can also talk about how you deal with something that frightens you and read stories about children who are afraid and conquer their fears.

- **Use imagination and be creative.** You can use your imagination to fight imaginary fears, such as that of monsters. Many families have found "monster spray" to be a wonderful way to help a child cope with bedtime fears. Take a spray-type bottle and fill it with water (be sure that it has not previously had any chemicals in it, such as plant food). At bedtime, you or your child can spray the room to keep the monsters away. In addition to monster spray, there are other ways in which you can be creative and help your child. For example, consider allowing him to have a pet for nighttime company. Even a bedside fish tank might help.
- **Introduce a security object.** Helping your child become attached to a security object that he can keep in bed with him may be beneficial. This may help your child to feel more relaxed throughout the night.
- **Use a nightlight.** No matter what your child is afraid of, a nightlight can help. A nightlight is fine as long as it does not prevent your child from falling asleep. Another thing to try is leaving the bedroom door open so that your child doesn't feel isolated from the rest of the family.
- **Avoid scary television shows.** Avoid scary TV shows, videos, or stories that may add to your child's fears.
- **Teach relaxation training.** Teaching your child relaxation strategies can help him relax at bedtime and fall asleep. This will give him something else to think about while lying in bed and help to distract him from his fearful thoughts. Also, it is impossible to be relaxed and scared at the same time.
- **Discuss your child's fears during the day.** Depending on how old your child is and how well he can talk, try discussing his fears during the day. Talk about how he can be less frightened at night. In addition, build his self-confidence during the day. Feeling secure throughout the day may help him feel more secure at night as well.
- **Set limits.** At the same time that you are reassuring your child, you need to set limits. Limits are necessary to prevent your child's "being scared" behavior from being reinforced. Checking closets and leaving a low nightlight on is reasonable, but sleeping with your child every night is not.
- **Have him stay in his bed.** Don't encourage your child to get out of bed. He should stay in bed and find out for himself that he really is safe so that he can learn to overcome his fears. If you bring your child into your room, or downstairs while finishing the dinner dishes, the message is that his bed isn't a safe place to be. It is a much better strategy to stay with him in *his* room than to have him join you in yours. If your child is too frightened to stay in his room alone, it is okay to *occasionally* stay by his bed until he falls asleep. Don't do this too frequently, or even for two nights in a row, because he may come to depend on your presence. If your child is anxious about your leaving, check on him frequently. Begin by briefly checking and reassuring him in 5 minutes, and then every 10 minutes until he is asleep. Similarly, if your child wakes up in the middle of the night and can't go back to sleep because he is frightened,

go and reassure him. Repeat the message about being safe and tell him that he will be fine. If he gets up in the middle of the night and comes into your room, take him right back and gently tuck him into bed. Reassure him again, but don't let him get up.

- **Start a star/sticker chart.** Some children receive reinforcement for their fears. They may be given lots of attention for being afraid or receive special treats. If this is the case, switch the scenario. Give your child extra attention for dealing with his fears. Tell him how proud you are of him for being brave. Set up a star system. Have him earn stars for being brave and sleeping on his own. After earning a certain number of stars, he can turn them in for a treat, such as watching a favorite video, going to the park, or baking cookies.
- **Address severe or persistent anxiety.** If your child's anxiety and fears continue, are severe, or are present during the day, consider taking him for a psychological evaluation aimed at identifying and treating anxiety.

Appendix F4

Nightmares

WHAT ARE NIGHTMARES?

Nightmares are scary dreams that can wake a child leaving her upset and in need of comfort. They are very common in children. It is rare to find someone who has never experienced a nightmare. After a nightmare, most children are afraid to go back to sleep and often do not want to be left alone. Very young children do not know the difference between a dream and reality, so when they wake up, they may not understand the concept that they were only dreaming and it is now over. They may keep insisting that something scary is about to occur.

What do children have nightmares about? Most young toddlers have concerns about being separated from their parents. So they may have a nightmare about being lost or having something happen to one of their parents. Nightmares also are more likely to happen following some difficult event in the child's life. For example, if a child has just started day care or if her parents have gone away overnight, she is more likely to have a nightmare. For young children, nightmares may also be the reliving of a traumatic event, such as getting lost, getting a shot at the doctors, or being barked at by a big dog. By age 2 years, nightmares begin to incorporate monsters and scary things that can hurt a child. Older children often have nightmares related to scary movies or stories or a frightening daytime experience.

WHAT CAUSES NIGHTMARES?

Nightmares are usually a part of normal development and are a sign of a young child's developing imagination. Children are also more likely to have nightmares after a frightening experience.

There are several things that you can do to help reduce the likelihood of nightmares:

• **Avoid scary stories, television shows, or movies before bedtime.** These will increase the likelihood of your child having a nightmare. Choose instead a comforting bedtime routine.

- **Identify stressors.** If there is something in your child's life that you know is distressing, try to take care of it and reassure your child. If your child suddenly experiences a significant increase in the frequency or intensity of nightmares, try to evaluate why. Look for recurring themes that could give you a clue as to the cause and then deal with the problem.
- **Ensure that your child is getting enough sleep.** Children are much more likely to have nightmares after not getting enough sleep. If your child is having nightmares, make sure that she is getting enough sleep as this can help decrease both the frequency and the intensity of nightmares.

HOW SHOULD YOU RESPOND TO YOUR CHILD'S NIGHTMARES?

If your child has a nightmare, there are a few things that you should do:

- **Offer reassurance.** The best thing that you can do if your child has a nightmare is comfort her. For babies and young toddlers, merely holding them and providing physical comfort is enough. For older children, verbal reassurance may also be needed. Following most nightmares, your child will be reassured by a few minutes of comfort. Stay with her in her room. Let her know that you are nearby and will make sure that she is safe and secure. Most children are still tired after a nightmare and will be ready to fall back to sleep.
- **Give your child a security object.** Helping a child become attached to a security object that she can keep in bed with her can be beneficial. This often helps a child feel more relaxed throughout the night.
- **Leave a light on.** If your child insists on having a light on, put it on the dimmest setting possible so that your child can fall back to sleep.
- **Discuss it the next day.** The next day, you may want to try and talk to your child about her nightmare to see if there is anything bothering her. Most of the time nightmares are isolated events with little meaning, but if your child starts having them on a frequent basis, you should try and figure out what is disturbing her.
- **Encourage the use of imagination.** Some children do well with using their imagination to get rid of nightmares. Your child can draw pictures of her bad dreams and then throw them away, or she can imagine different endings to her nightmares. Even a dream catcher hung over her bed may be reassuring.
- **Get outside help.** If your child's nightmares are severe, meaning that they are interfering in her life or occurring on a very frequent basis, speak to her physician or a mental health provider.

Appendix F5

Sleepwalking

WHAT IS SLEEPWALKING?

Sleepwalking is a benign (not harmful) sleep behavior that is common in children. A sleepwalking child may have his eyes open, but usually appears confused or dazed during an episode, and mumbles or gives inappropriate answers to questions. Occasionally, a sleepwalking child may appear agitated. A sleepwalker is often clumsy and may perform bizarre or strange actions, such as urinating in a closet. Sleepwalking almost always occurs within 1–2 hours after falling asleep, lasts from 5 to 20 minutes, and children have no memory of these events. Although a child sleepwalking may appear awake, he is really asleep. Sleepwalking can occur infrequently or every night.

WHAT CAUSES SLEEPWALKING?

We do not know what exactly causes sleepwalking, but it is very common in childhood. Almost 40% of all children will sleepwalk at some time, with peak occurrence between 3 and 7 years. Sleepwalking often runs in families and most children outgrow it by adolescence. Sleepwalking can also be associated with night terrors.

There are certain things that make it more likely for someone who is prone to sleepwalking to have an episode. These include:

- Not getting enough sleep
- An irregular sleep schedule
- Fever, illness
- Some medications
- Sleeping with a full bladder
- Sleeping in a different environment
- Noisy sleeping environment
- Stress

HOW SHOULD YOU RESPOND TO YOUR CHILD'S SLEEPWALKING?

- **Keep your child safe.** Sleepwalkers can injure themselves or leave the house during an episode. Make sure that all outside doors and windows are secure. The sleeping environment should be made as safe as possible to avoid accidental injury. Floors should not be cluttered, objects should not be left on the stairs, and hallways should be lit. Tying bells to your child's bedroom door can alert you to the sleepwalking incident. Some parents keep their sleepwalker confined to the bedroom by securely fashioning a screen door or high gate to the bedroom door.
- **Guide your child back to bed.** Guide your child gently back to bed while speaking to him in a calm and soothing manner.
- **Don't wake your child.** Generally, nothing is gained by trying to wake a sleepwalking child, and it may even make your child more agitated. However, nothing bad will happen if he does awaken.
- **Ensure enough sleep.** Increase the amount of sleep that your child is getting and try to not let him become sleep deprived. Sleepwalking is much more likely to happen when your child does not get enough sleep.
- **Maintain a regular sleep schedule.** Sleepwalking is more likely to happen on nights when your child goes to sleep at a different time than usual.
- **Additional treatment.** In most cases, sleepwalking requires no treatment. However, in cases in which a child is at risk for harm or sleepwalking is occurring frequently, treatment may be necessary. Treatment may include medication or behavior modification techniques. Be sure to speak to your child's doctor if you are concerned.

Appendix F6

Sleep Terrors

WHAT ARE SLEEP TERRORS?

Sleep terrors, or night terrors as they are often called, are dramatic and can be distressing to witness. A child having a sleep terror may have her eyes open but usually appears very agitated, frightened and even panicked, as well as confused and dazed during an episode. A child will often cry out or scream at the beginning of the sleep terror and may mumble or give inappropriate answers to questions. A child having a sleep terror is often clumsy and may flail around, push a parent away, or behave in other strange ways. As disturbing and frightening as these events appear to the observer, children having them usually are totally unaware of what they are doing. In fact, sleep terrors are much worse to watch than to experience. For the child, a sleep terror is less traumatic than a typical nightmare or bad dream.

Sleep terrors almost always occur within 1–2 hours after falling asleep, last anywhere from a few minutes to an hour, and children have no memory of these events (note that sleep terrors can also occur during a nap). In addition, during these events most children avoid being comforted. They may get more upset if you talk to them and try to calm them down. This can be the hardest part for parents. Although a child having a sleep terror may appear awake, she is really asleep. A child who is experiencing a sleep terror is basically stuck halfway between asleep and awake.

Finally, sleep terrors are not nightmares. Your child is not dreaming during these events, although it may look it. Sleep terrors are also not a sign of psychological problems or the result of a traumatic event.

WHAT CAUSES SLEEP TERRORS?

Sleep terrors are benign (not harmful) sleep behaviors, but they may cause a great deal of anxiety for parents. We do not know what exactly causes sleep terrors or why children look frightened during them. They are actually the same thing as sleepwalking, but just more dramatic.

Sleep terrors are fairly common in children and usually occur in preschool-aged and elementary school–aged children. Most children outgrow sleep terrors by adolescence. In addition, sleep terrors and sleepwalking often run in families.

There are certain things that make it more likely for someone who is prone to sleep terrors to have an episode. These include:

- Not getting enough sleep
- An irregular sleep schedule
- Fever, illness
- Some medications
- Sleeping with a full bladder
- Sleeping in a different environment
- Sleeping in a noisy environment
- Stress

HOW SHOULD YOU RESPOND TO YOUR CHILD'S SLEEP TERRORS?

- **Keep your child safe.** The most important thing that you can do if your child has sleep terrors is to keep her safe. Make sure that all outside doors are secure. Put up gates at the door of your child's bedroom and at the top of stairs. An alarm can signal you when your child is up and about, and help to ensure that she does not leave the house. Any type of alarm will do, from a fancy and expensive burglar alarm to a simple bell hung on the door. Ensure that windows, especially second story or higher, do not open wide enough that your child can jump out of them. Finally, remove things that are in the way. If your child may walk or run around during a sleep terror, clear away anything that she can step on or trip over.
- **Don't wake your child.** Generally, nothing is gained by trying to awaken a child during a sleep terror, and sometimes doing so can make a child more agitated.
- **Guide your child back to bed.** To encourage return to normal sleep, guide your child gently back to bed. If she resists, let her be.
- **Try not to interfere too much.** The normal response of parents is to try and comfort their child during one of these episodes. Try to resist doing this. Most children will just get more agitated. However, if your child is about to come to harm, be sure to keep her safe even if she fights you.
- **Ensure enough sleep.** Increase the amount of sleep that your child is getting and try to let not let her become sleep deprived. These events are much more likely to happen when your child does not get enough sleep.
- **Maintain a regular sleep schedule.** Sleep terrors are more likely to happen on nights when your child goes to sleep at a different time than usual.
- **Don't discuss sleep terrors the next day.** The morning after an event, do not make a point of discussing the episode with your child. Discussing the event is likely to worry her. However, if she brings it up, simply reassure her.

- **Additional treatment.** In most cases, sleep terrors require no treatment. However, in severe cases, when these behaviors involve injury, violence, or serious disruption to the family, treatment may be necessary. Treatment may include medication or behavior modification techniques. Be sure to speak to your child's doctor if your child has frequent or severe sleep terrors and you are concerned.

Appendix F7

Headbanging and Bodyrocking

WHAT IS HEADBANGING?

Headbanging and bodyrocking are officially called rhythmic movement disorders. Rhythmic movement disorder usually involves some type of rocking, rolling, or headbanging. Oddly, children find this a soothing way to fall asleep. Your child probably does this most times that he is falling asleep, whether at naptime or bedtime. Furthermore, given that all children naturally wake frequently during the night, your child will need to headbang (or rock) to put himself back to sleep in the middle of the night. So don't be surprised that this behavior occurs not only at bedtime but throughout the night.

SHOULD YOU BE CONCERNED ABOUT YOUR CHILD'S HEADBANGING OR BODYROCKING?

For almost all children, headbanging or bodyrocking is of no concern. It is a common way to fall asleep. There are some children for whom it may be of concern, though. Some children with other issues, such as developmental delay, autism, or blindness, will rock or bang their heads, and may hurt themselves. This type of behavior is substantially different and will occur both throughout the day and at night. If your child is normal and healthy during the day and only bangs his head to fall asleep, you should not be concerned. Also, if your child has a neurological or psychiatric problem, you will likely be aware of it from his behavior during the day.

HOW SHOULD YOU RESPOND TO YOUR CHILD'S HEADBANGING OR BODYROCKING?

There is nothing much that you need to do if your child headbangs or rocks himself to sleep. Children often rock or bang their heads to fall asleep. This is normal. Most will eventually stop by 4 years of age. In the meantime, there are some things to consider:

- **Don't worry about trying to protect your child.** Even if your child is banging his head hard, it is unlikely that he will hurt himself. Thus, there is no need to put extra bumpers on the crib or place pillows in strategic places. Also, it rarely works. Most children will find a way to bang their heads, no matter what creative tricks you try.

- **Be careful not to reinforce the headbanging.** If you go in to your child every time he starts to rock or bang his head, you may be reinforcing his behavior without even realizing it. In this case, he may be headbanging to get your attention. Make sure that your child gets lots of attention during the day and ignore his headbanging at night.
- **Move the crib or bed.** Move the crib or the bed away from the wall if the banging or rocking is making noise and keeping the rest of the family awake. If your child is in a bed rather than a crib, put guardrails on all sides, so he won't fall out of bed. If our child is making his crib or bed squeak, oil the screws and bolts.
- **Ensure your child's safety.** Be sure to tighten all screws and bolts on your child's crib or bed on a regular basis, as the rocking or headbanging can loosen them.

Appendix F8

Bruxism

WHAT IS BRUXISM?

Bruxism is the medical term for teethgrinding. Surprisingly, teeth grinding is common in children. Children and adolescents can grind their teeth in any stage of sleep but are more likely to do it during the first half of the night, when non-REM sleep is more common. However, some individuals only grind their teeth during REM sleep (dreaming sleep), which mostly occurs in the second half of the night.

TEETHGRINDING IN BABIES

Almost 50% of babies grind their teeth. It usually begins at about age 10 months, after the baby has her deciduous incisors (the two top front teeth and the two bottom front teeth). Some babies only grind their teeth sporadically, whereas others can do it throughout most of the night. In babies, teeth grinding is not of any concern and eventually goes away on its own. While teeth grinding in adults can lead to dental problems, teeth grinding in babies is nothing to be alarmed about. It is highly unlikely that a child is doing any damage to her teeth. However, if the teeth grinding is worrisome or if there are any changes in your child's teeth, do see a dentist. Some babies are less likely to grind their teeth while lying on their side, so you can try turning a baby and putting her on her side to fall asleep or once she is asleep.

TEETHGRINDING IN CHILDREN AND ADOLESCENTS

Bruxism also occurs in older children and adolescents, usually beginning after age 10 years. Almost 95% of all adults have ground their teeth at least once in their life, and many do it often. It is seen just as often in children. Teeth grinding is also more common in children with disabilities, especially those with cerebral palsy and mental retardation. In addition to teeth grinding, other symptoms may include teeth pain, temporomandibular joint pain, and headaches. Furthermore, dental erosion can be a concern with frequent bruxism. Finally, stress is likely to result in increased bruxism.

WHAT YOU CAN DO ABOUT BRUXISM

Nothing much needs to be done if a child is grinding her teeth. It is usually of little concern. However, relaxation strategies may be helpful. Furthermore, if a child is experiencing headaches, having tooth pain, or is wearing down her teeth, an evaluation by a dentist is warranted. Older children and adolescents may benefit from a mouth guard, which prevents dental erosion.

Appendix F9

Obstructive Sleep Apnea in Children

WHAT IS OBSTRUCTIVE SLEEP APNEA?

Obstructive sleep apnea is a medical condition in which a child has repeated, brief, temporary breathing pauses (apneas) during sleep. Lack of breathing causes a decrease in oxygen and an increase in carbon dioxide (CO_2) in the body. These changes signal the brain that breathing has stopped; the brain then signals the body to briefly awaken and restart breathing.

Thus, these obstructions result in frequent brief arousals from sleep. Although the actual number of minutes of arousal during the night may be small, these repeated, brief disruptions in sleep could lead to significant daytime symptoms in children. A comparable image would be that of being poked by someone 15–30 times a night. However, children are usually unaware of waking up, and parents often describe very restless sleep but usually do not say that their child wakes up completely.

WHAT CAUSES OBSTRUCTIVE SLEEP APNEA?

In most children, sleep apnea is caused by large tonsils and/or adenoids, which can block the airway. Sleep apnea is also more common in children who are overweight, although some children with enlarged tonsils and/or adenoids may be underweight. Younger children with sleep apnea may have poor growth because of disruption in nighttime secretion of growth hormone. Other children who are at high risk for sleep apnea include those with a narrow facial bone structure, a history of cleft palate, and Down syndrome. Children with allergies, asthma, reflux, or frequent sinus infections may also be at risk for obstructive sleep apnea.

WHAT ARE THE SYMPTOMS OF OBSTRUCTIVE SLEEP APNEA?

- Snoring
- Breathing pauses during sleep or difficulty breathing during sleep
- Mouth breathing
- Noisy breathing
- Restless sleep
- Sweating during sleep
- Morning headaches
- Difficulty waking in the morning
- Nasal voice

Children with obstructive sleep apnea may also have daytime symptoms as a result of the sleep disruption. They may be sleepy during the day, taking unplanned naps or falling asleep in school. Children with sleep apnea may also be moody, irritable, or cranky. In addition, behavior problems and poor school performance may be noted.

HOW IS OBSTRUCTIVE SLEEP APNEA DIAGNOSED?

Many children with symptoms of obstructive sleep apnea require an overnight sleep study to confirm the diagnosis. The overnight sleep study, which is done in a specialized sleep laboratory, monitors breathing, heart rate, and sleep interruptions.

HOW IS OBSTRUCTIVE SLEEP APNEA TREATED?

For most children with sleep apnea, removal of tonsils and adenoids, if enlarged, takes care of the problem. An ear, nose, and throat specialist makes the evaluation for such surgery. Children who are overweight should be counseled about nutrition and exercise. Those with allergies or asthma may be treated with medication. Nasal sprays or sleeping in positions in which the child does not snore may also be recommended. Some children require a treatment called continuous positive airway pressure, which is a portable breathing machine used at night.

Appendix F10

Restless Legs Syndrome

WHAT IS RESTLESS LEGS SYNDROME?

Restless legs syndrome is a movement disorder in which a child or adolescent experiences uncomfortable sensations in the legs during periods of rest or sitting still. The sensations are usually described as creepy, crawly, tingling, or painful. Some parents interpret their child's complaints as "growing pains." To relieve the discomfort, children or adolescents with restless legs syndrome will likely have an overwhelming urge to move their legs, whether stretching them, getting up and walking or running around, or simply tossing and turning. In addition, rubbing the legs may make them feel better. Because of the leg discomfort and increased leg movements, it often takes a long time for a child or adolescent with restless legs syndrome to fall asleep at bedtime.

A second sleep disorder that often goes along with restless legs syndrome is periodic limb movement disorder (PLMD). This is also a movement disorder in which the legs kick or twitch during sleep. Unlike restless legs syndrome, a child with PLMD is usually not aware of the symptoms, although a parent may observe kicking and restless sleep. The only symptom may be daytime fatigue that is a result of the disturbed sleep.

WHAT CAUSES RESTLESS LEGS SYNDROME?

The cause of restless legs syndrome is unknown. It can run in families, and thus, there is likely a genetic basis to some cases. Restless legs syndrome can also be related to low iron (anemia). In addition, some children with chronic diseases, such as diabetes and kidney disease, are at increased risk for developing restless legs syndrome.

WHAT ARE THE SYMPTOMS OF RESTLESS LEGS SYNDROME?

The symptoms of restless legs syndrome include:

- **Leg discomfort.** Children or adolescents often describe these uncomfortable leg sensations as creepy, crawly, painful, or tingling. These sensations usually occur at bedtime but can also occur at other times of inactivity, such as during long car rides or while watching a movie.
- **Leg movements.** To relieve the leg discomfort, children and adolescents with restless legs syndrome often have an irresistible urge to move their legs, whether by tossing and turning while lying in bed, or by walking or running about at bedtime.
- **Sleep disruption.** Children and adolescents with restless legs syndrome often take a long time to fall asleep because of the leg discomfort and need to move. They not only have problems falling asleep but may also have difficulty staying asleep.
- **Bedtime behavior problems.** Because of the difficulty with falling asleep, parents may report that their child is a problem at bedtime due to not staying in bed.
- **Daytime sleepiness.** The difficulties falling asleep and staying asleep can result in significant daytime sleepiness.
- **Behavior and academic problems.** Children and adolescents with restless legs syndrome may have daytime behavior and academic problems, such as hyperactivity, impulsivity, and irritability, which is the result of the sleep disruption.

HOW IS RESTLESS LEGS SYNDROME DIAGNOSED?

There is no definitive test for restless legs syndrome, so diagnosis is made based on the description of symptoms. A medical history and physical examination will also be done to exclude other problems. Finally, an overnight sleep study may be recommended to evaluate for other sleep disorders, especially PLMD.

HOW IS RESTLESS LEGS SYNDROME TREATED?

Treatment for restless legs syndrome may involve any of the following:

- **Change bedtime habits.** Given that the leg discomfort gets worse the longer the child or adolescent lies in bed, it is usually better for the child to wait to get into bed until she is ready to turn out the light. Therefore, the bedtime routine, such as reading stories, should all occur out of bed.

- **Avoid caffeine.** Caffeine can make restless legs syndrome symptoms worse; so all caffeine should be avoided. Caffeine can be found in many sodas, tea, and coffee, but also in chocolate and medications (e.g., Midol, Excedrin).
- **Reduce the discomfort.** Massage, cold compresses, or a heating pad may provide temporary relief.
- **Rule out iron deficiency.** Low levels of iron or folic acid can contribute to restless legs syndrome symptoms, so an iron or folic acid supplement may be prescribed.
- **Consider medication.** For children and adolescents with restless legs syndrome who have significant sleep disruption, medication may be recommended. There are a number of different types of medications that can help.

Appendix F11

Periodic Limb Movement Disorder

WHAT IS PERIODIC LIMB MOVEMENT DISORDER?

Periodic limb movement disorder (PLMD) involves periodic episodes of repetitive movements, usually in the legs, that occur approximately every 20 to 40 seconds. The movements may appear as brief muscle twitches, jerking movements, or an upward flexing of the feet. These movements occur in clusters, lasting from a few minutes to a few hours. Most children and adolescents with PLMD are not aware of the movements. PLMD can result in frequent brief arousals throughout the night, leading to daytime sleepiness.

Children and adolescents with PLMD may also have restless legs syndrome, a movement disorder in which an individual experiences uncomfortable sensations in the legs during periods of rest or sitting still. The sensations are usually described as creepy, crawly, tingling, or painful and can make it difficult for a child or adolescent to fall asleep at bedtime.

WHAT CAUSES PERIODIC LIMB MOVEMENT DISORDER?

The cause of PLMD is unknown, but it may be related to low iron (anemia). In addition, some children with chronic diseases, such as diabetes and kidney disease, are at increased risk for developing PLMD.

WHAT ARE THE SYMPTOMS OF PERIODIC LIMB MOVEMENT DISORDER?

The symptoms of PLMD may include any of the following, although many children and adolescents with the condition do not report any symptoms:

* **Leg movements.** Repetitive leg movements in sleep characterize PLMD, but the child or adolescent is probably not aware of these movements.

- **Sleep disruption.** Children and adolescents with PLMD may experience wakings throughout the night as a result of the multiple arousals from sleep.
- **Restless sleep.** A child or adolescent with PLMD may be described as a restless sleeper due to the leg movements and frequent arousals.
- **Daytime sleepiness.** The frequent arousals in sleep can result in significant daytime sleepiness.
- **Behavior and academic problems.** Children and adolescents with PLMD may have daytime behavior and academic problems, such as hyperactivity, impulsivity, and irritability, which is the result of the sleep disruption.

HOW IS PERIODIC LIMB MOVEMENT DISORDER DIAGNOSED?

PLMD is diagnosed by an overnight sleep study. This requires your child or adolescent to stay overnight in a sleep laboratory. In addition, a medical history and physical examination will be conducted.

HOW IS PERIODIC LIMB MOVEMENT DISORDER TREATED?

Treatment for PLMD may involve any of the following:

- **Use of medication.** For children and adolescents with PLMD who have significant sleep disruption, medication may be recommended. There are a number of different medications that can help.
- **Avoidance of caffeine.** Caffeine can make PLMD symptoms worse; so all caffeine should be avoided. Caffeine can be found in many sodas, tea, and coffee, but also in chocolate and medications (e.g., Midol, Excedrin).
- **Management of iron deficiency.** Low levels of iron or folic acid can contribute to PLMD symptoms, so an iron or folic acid supplement may be prescribed by your child's doctor.

Appendix F12

Narcolepsy

WHAT IS NARCOLEPSY?

Narcolepsy is a chronic (lifelong) neurologic (affecting the brain or nerves) disorder that is characterized by a permanent and overwhelming feeling of sleepiness. Narcolepsy affects more than 1 in 2,000 Americans, and most cases go undiagnosed and untreated. Although it is a relatively uncommon condition, its impact on a child's life can be dramatic. It affects boys and girls equally, and symptoms usually develop after puberty, with most people reporting the first symptoms of narcolepsy between the ages of 15 and 30.

WHAT ARE THE SYMPTOMS OF NARCOLEPSY?

The symptoms of narcolepsy can appear all at once, or they can develop slowly over many years. The four most common symptoms are excessive day-time sleepiness, cataplexy, sleep paralysis, and hypnagogic hallucinations. In some cases, excessive daytime sleepiness is the only symptom.

- **Excessive daytime sleepiness** is usually the first symptom of narcolepsy. People with narcolepsy often report feeling tired all the time. They tend to fall asleep not only in situations in which many normal people feel sleepy (after meals or during a dull lecture), but also when most people would remain awake (while watching a movie or writing a letter). Individuals with narcolepsy may also fall asleep at unusual times (in the middle of a conversation) or dangerous times (driving a car).
- **Cataplexy** involves sudden, brief losses of muscle control triggered by stress or a strong emotion, such as laughter, anger, or surprise. Cataplexy can range from a brief feeling of weakness in the knees to complete collapse. Cataplexy is sometimes the first symptom of narcolepsy but usually develops several years after the daytime sleepiness.
- **Sleep paralysis** is a feeling of being paralyzed, including being unable to talk or move for a brief period, either when falling asleep or after waking up. Touching the person usually causes the paralysis to disappear.

- **Hypnagogic hallucinations** are vivid, dream-like experiences that are difficult to distinguish from reality, occurring at sleep onset or after awakening. The images are often scary, such as of strange animals or prowlers, and are particularly frightening because the child is awake but has no control over the action.

A child or adolescent with narcolepsy may also have other symptoms:

- **Automatic behavior** is the performance of familiar, routine, or boring tasks without full awareness or later memory of doing them. Sometimes a child may actually fall asleep and continue an activity, but not recall having done it when awakened. Examples of automatic behavior include writing a letter or doing homework.
- **Disturbed nighttime sleep** frequently occurs in children and adolescents with narcolepsy. Although they have difficulty staying awake during the day, they may also wake frequently during the night. These multiple nighttime awakenings make the daytime sleepiness even worse.
- **Other symptoms** reported by children and adolescents with narcolepsy include lethargy, low motivation, inability to concentrate, and memory loss. Children often have problems in school and keeping up with friends.

WHAT CAUSES NARCOLEPSY?

Although narcolepsy has been extensively studied, its exact cause is not known. Narcolepsy appears to be a disorder of the part of the central nervous system that controls sleep and wakefulness. Cataplexy, sleep paralysis, and hypnagogic hallucinations are similar to the loss of muscle tone that accompanies a stage of sleep called REM (rapid eye movement) sleep. Narcolepsy often runs in families, but many people with narcolepsy do not have relatives who are affected. Narcolepsy is not caused by psychiatric or psychological problems.

HOW IS NARCOLEPSY DIAGNOSED?

Narcolepsy is usually diagnosed by medical history and an overnight sleep study. The next day following the sleep study, a multiple sleep latency test will also be done. This test evaluates for daytime sleepiness and involves taking four or five naps every 2 hours. The length of time needed to fall asleep and whether REM sleep occurs is recorded.

HOW IS NARCOLEPSY TREATED?

Narcolepsy cannot be cured, but its symptoms can usually be controlled so that a child or adolescent with narcolepsy can lead a normal life. Each treatment plan usually involves medication, life-style changes, and education.

- **Medication.** One or more medications are usually prescribed to control the excessive daytime sleepiness and cataplexy. Caffeine should be avoided, especially in the late afternoon and evening, so that nighttime sleep is not disturbed.
- **Lifestyle changes.** The effective treatment of narcolepsy requires not only medication but also adjustments in lifestyle. The following suggestions can bring substantial improvement:
  1. Follow a strict sleep–wake schedule that ensures adequate sleep. Your child should go to bed and get up at the same time each day.
  2. Take scheduled short naps once or twice each day, as needed.
  3. Increase physical activity; avoid boring or repetitive tasks.
  4. Avoid activities that can be dangerous, such as driving, swimming, or cooking, except during times when you know your child will be alert.
- **Education.** Narcolepsy can be a devastating disorder if family, friends, and teachers do not understand it, so education is essential. Daytime sleepiness may be mistaken for laziness, boredom, or lack of ability. The experiences of cataplexy and dreaming during wakefulness may be wrongly seen as a psychiatric problem. Be sure to educate family members and help your child's friends and their parents understand narcolepsy. Most importantly, make sure your child's teachers understand the disorder. Small adjustments in the classroom, such as being seated in the front of the class and being chosen to run classroom errands, can make a tremendous difference in a child's academic performance.

Appendix F13

Delayed Sleep Phase Syndrome

WHAT IS DELAYED SLEEP PHASE SYNDROME?

Delayed sleep phase syndrome (DSPS) is a disorder in which the person's sleep–wake cycle (internal clock) is delayed by 2 or more hours. Basically, it is a shift of the internal clock by 2 or more hours, in that sleep is postponed. For example, rather than falling asleep at 10 PM and waking at 7 AM, an adolescent with DSPS will not fall asleep until 12 AM or later and then has great difficulty awakening at 7 AM for school or work. If the child or adolescent is allowed to sleep until late in the morning, he will feel rested and can function well. Most children and adolescents with DSPS describe themselves as "night owls" and usually feel and function their best in the evening and nighttime hours. They usually get much less sleep on weekdays than on weekends or holidays.

Having DSPS, especially for children and adolescents who attend school, can cause significant problems, as they are unable to get up for school, often resulting in multiple school absences and tardiness.

WHAT CAUSES DELAYED SLEEP PHASE SYNDROME?

Delayed sleep phase syndrome usually develops during adolescence but can start in childhood. It seldom occurs after the age of 30. Although the cause of DSPS is not completely known, it likely is an exaggerated reaction to the normal shift in sleep times that occurs during adolescence. All adolescents have a shift in their internal clock after puberty of about 2 hours. In those with DSPS, the clock shifts even more. In addition, for children who already had a tendency to go to bed late, this normal 2-hour shift results in a significantly shifted internal clock. It is important to realize that this shift in sleep is not caused by deliberate behavior. Unfortunately, many adolescents with DSPS get labeled as noncompliant and truants. Approximately 7% of adolescents have DSPS; thus, it is a common disorder.

WHAT ARE THE SYMPTOMS OF DELAYED SLEEP PHASE SYNDROME?

A child or adolescent with DSPS often experiences the following symptoms:

- **Daytime sleepiness.** Because of the late sleep-onset times and the usual requirement to get up earlier than desired for school or work, children and adolescents with DSPS often experience daytime sleepiness as the result of not getting enough sleep.
- **Inability to fall asleep at the desired time.** On nights that children or adolescents with DSPS try to go to sleep at a "normal" time, they are unable to do so. However, if they were to go to bed at their usual fall-asleep time, they would have no problem falling asleep.
- **Inability to wake up at the desired time.** As a result of the late sleep-onset time, many children and adolescents with DSPS are unable to wake up in the morning for school or other activities. This can result in many absences or latenesses.
- **No other sleep complaints.** Because the internal clock is simply shifted in children and adolescents with DSPS, once asleep they sleep well with few or no awakenings. In addition, on days that they are able to sleep as long as they wish, especially on weekends or holidays, sleep is normal, and daytime sleepiness is not experienced.
- **Other daytime symptoms.** Some children and adolescents with DSPS experience problems with depression and other behavior problems as a result of the daytime sleepiness and the effects of missing school and social activities. In addition, there are a percentage of children and adolescents with DSPS who have school refusal, which complicates both diagnosis and treatment.

HOW IS DELAYED SLEEP PHASE SYNDROME DIAGNOSED?

There is no definitive test for DSPS, so the diagnosis is made based on a description of the problem. An overnight sleep study may be recommended to ensure that no other sleep disorder is present, such as obstructive sleep apnea or restless legs syndrome.

HOW IS DELAYED SLEEP PHASE SYNDROME TREATED?

Delayed sleep phase syndrome is a difficult disorder to treat and requires significant effort on the part of the child or adolescent. Thus, for treatment to be successful, the child or adolescent has to be very motivated. The goal of treatment is to retrain the internal clock to a more regular schedule. However, making the initial shift in the sleep–wake cycle is easier than maintaining that change. Treatment can involve the following:

- **Sleep hygiene.** Good sleep habits are especially important for children and adolescents with DSPS. These habits should include a regular sleep schedule that encompasses going to bed and waking up at the same time every day; avoidance of caffeine, smoking, and other drugs; a bedroom environment that is cool, quiet, and comfortable; a bedtime routine that is calm and sleep inducing; and avoidance of all stimulating activities before bed, such as computer games and television.
- **Shifting the internal clock.** Treatment for DSPS involves systematically advancing or delaying bedtime on successive nights.
  - **Phase advancement.** Phase advancement involves moving the bedtime earlier by 15 minutes on successive nights. If the adolescent usually falls asleep at 12:30, then bedtime is set for 12:15 for one or two nights, 12:00 for one to two nights, and so on.
  - **Phase delay (chronotherapy).** Phase delay is chosen if the adolescent's naturally occurring bedtime is 3 or more hours later than desired. Bedtime is delayed by 2 to 3 hours on successive nights. For example, if an adolescent usually falls asleep at 2 AM, bedtime is delayed until 4 AM on night one, 6 AM on night two, and so on until the desired bedtime is reached (e.g., 10:30 PM). Given that it is much easier for the body to adjust to a later bedtime than an earlier one, it is often recommended to delay bedtime rather than try to advance it.
  - **Sticking with it.** Once the desired bedtime is reached, the adolescent must stick with it on a nightly basis. Even one night of late-night studying or socializing can return the internal clock to the delayed state. However, usually after several months the schedule can become a bit more flexible.
- **Bright-light therapy.** Sometimes bright-light therapy is recommended, which involves exposing the child to bright light in the morning for approximately 20 to 30 minutes, and avoiding bright light in the evening. Bright light in the morning helps to reset the body's internal clock. Special light boxes must be purchased for this treatment.

Appendix F14

Insomnia

WHAT IS INSOMNIA?

Insomnia refers to difficulties with falling asleep or staying asleep, including the problem of waking too early in the morning. It is one of the most common sleep complaints made by adults, but is much less prevalent in children and adolescents. Insomnia can be a short-term problem, usually related to a stressful event, or it can be long-term and chronic.

Many times, insomnia is a symptom that is caused by another sleep disorder. Just like pain, which can be a symptom of many things, problems with falling asleep or staying asleep may be the result of another sleep disorder or other problem (e.g., anxiety). When the insomnia is not related to another sleep disturbance, psychiatric problem, or medical problem, it is referred to as primary insomnia or psychophysiologic insomnia.

WHAT CAUSES INSOMNIA?

Primary insomnia almost always involves (a) poor sleep habits, such as spending too much time in bed, napping during the day, or not going to bed and waking up at the same time every day and (b) negative thoughts about sleep, such as "I'll never be able to fall asleep tonight."

WHAT ARE THE SYMPTOMS OF INSOMNIA?

A child or adolescent with insomnia may have the following symptoms:

- **Sleep problems.** A child or adolescent with insomnia has difficulty falling asleep or staying asleep, or may wake too early in the morning.
- **Behaviors that interfere with sleep.** Such behaviors may include (a) worrying during the day about falling asleep at night and (b) trying too hard to fall asleep. (But adolescents with insomnia usually can fall asleep at other times, such as while watching television).

- **Tension about sleep.** A child or adolescent with insomnia is usually tense about going to bed and about being able to sleep.
- **Daytime problems.** A child or adolescent with insomnia may complain about having difficulty functioning during the day, is often tired, and may be moody or irritable.

HOW IS INSOMNIA DIAGNOSED?

There is no definitive test for insomnia, so a diagnosis is made based on the description of symptoms. A medical history should also be done to exclude other problems, such as another sleep disorder, a medical problem, or a psychiatric problem.

HOW IS INSOMNIA TREATED?

Treatment of insomnia, because it is a learned habit, requires effort and patience. Treatment can involve the following:

- **Sleep hygiene.** Good sleep habits are essential for children and adolescents with insomnia. These habits should include a regular sleep schedule that involves going to bed and waking up at the same time every day; avoiding caffeine, tobacco, and other drugs; sleeping in a room that is cool, quiet, and comfortable; establishing a bedtime routine that is calm and sleep inducing; and avoiding all stimulating activities at or close to bedtime, such as computer games and television.
- **Relaxation.** Teaching a child or adolescent relaxation strategies, such as deep breathing, positive imagery (e.g., being on a beach), or meditation, can help her to relax at bedtime. It will also give her something pleasant to think about while lying in bed.
- **Change thoughts about sleep.** Since most children or adolescents with insomnia have negative thoughts about sleep, such thoughts should be replaced by positive ones. For example, rather than saying, "I won't be able to sleep tonight," it is better to think, "Tonight I'll just relax and rest at bedtime."
- **Don't be a clock watcher.** Remove the clock from the bedroom, as watching a clock during the night may feed your child's anxiety, thus making it harder for her to fall asleep.
- **Restrict the time in bed.** Set bedtime so that the time in bed is equal to the usual amount of sleep each night, such as 7 or 8 hours. Being extra sleepy will help a child or adolescent to fall asleep right away and stay asleep. Once that happens, bedtime can be moved earlier by 15 minutes every few nights until the desired bedtime is reached.
- **Get out of bed.** Rather than lying in bed tossing and turning, it's better to get out of bed and do another activity, which will also help prevent the bedroom from being associated with sleeplessness. After 20 minutes of trying to fall

asleep, get out of bed for 20 minutes and do something relaxing (such as reading, not watching television!). Then try again, repeating the 20 minutes in bed, 20 minutes out of bed cycle.

- **Medication.** Medications are usually not recommended for children and adolescents with insomnia.

Appendix F15

Sleep Tips for Children

The following recommendations will help your child get the best sleep possible and make it easier for him or her to fall asleep and stay asleep:

- **Sleep schedule.** Your child's bedtime and wake-up time should be about the same time everyday. There should not be more than an hour's difference in bedtime and wake-up time between school nights and nonschool nights.
- **Bedtime routine.** Your child should have a 20- to 30-minute bedtime routine that is the same every night. The routine should include calm activities, such as reading a book or talking about the day, with the last part occurring in the room where your child sleeps.
- **Bedroom.** Your child's bedroom should be comfortable, quiet, and dark. A nightlight is fine, as a completely dark room can be scary for some children. Your child will sleep better in a room that is cool (less than 75°F). Also, avoid using your child's bedroom for time out or other punishment. You want your child to think of the bedroom as a good place, not a bad one.
- **Snack.** Your child should not go to bed hungry. A light snack (such as milk and cookies) before bed is a good idea. Heavy meals within an hour or two of bedtime, however, may interfere with sleep.
- **Caffeine.** Your child should avoid caffeine for at least 3 to 4 hours before bedtime. Caffeine can be found in many types of soda, coffee, iced tea, and chocolate.
- **Evening activities.** The hour before bed should be a quiet time. Your child should not get involved in high-energy activities, such as rough play or playing outside, or stimulating activities, such as computer games.
- **Television.** Keep the television set out of your child's bedroom. Children can easily develop the bad habit of "needing" the television to fall asleep. It is also much more difficult to control your child's television viewing if the set is in the bedroom.
- **Naps.** Naps should be geared to your child's age and developmental needs. However, very long naps or too many naps should be avoided, as too much daytime sleep can result in your child sleeping less at night.
- **Exercise.** Your child should spend time outside every day and get daily exercise.

Appendix F16

Sleep Tips for Adolescents

The following recommendations will help you get the best sleep possible and make it easier for you to fall asleep and stay asleep:

- **Sleep schedule.** Wake up and go to bed at about the same time on school nights and nonschool nights. Bedtime and wake time should not differ from one day to the next by more than an hour or so.
- **Weekends.** Don't sleep in on weekends to "catch up" on sleep. This makes it more likely that you will have problems falling asleep at bedtime.
- **Naps.** If you are very sleepy during the day, nap for 30 to 45 minutes in the early afternoon. Don't nap too long or too late in the afternoon or you will have difficulty falling asleep at bedtime.
- **Sunlight.** Spend time outside every day, especially in the morning, as exposure to sunlight, or bright light, helps to keep your body's internal clock on track.
- **Exercise.** Exercise regularly. Exercising may help you fall asleep and sleep more deeply.
- **Bedroom.** Make sure your bedroom is comfortable, quiet, and dark. Make sure also that it is not too warm at night, as sleeping in a room warmer than 75°F will make it hard to sleep.
- **Bed.** Use your bed only for sleeping. Don't study, read, or listen to music on your bed.
- **Bedtime.** Make the 30 to 60 minutes before bedtime a quiet or wind-down time. Relaxing, calm, enjoyable activities, such as reading a book or listening to soothing music, help your body and mind slow down enough to let you sleep. Do not watch TV, study, exercise, or get involved in "energizing" activities in the 30 minutes before bedtime.
- **Snack.** Eat regular meals and don't go to bed hungry. A light snack before bed is a good idea; eating a full meal in the hour before bed is not.
- **Caffeine.** Avoid eating or drinking products containing caffeine in the late afternoon and evening. These include caffeinated sodas, coffee, tea, and chocolate.

- **Alcohol.** Ingestion of alcohol disrupts sleep and may cause you to awaken throughout the night.
- **Smoking.** Smoking disturbs sleep. Don't smoke for at least an hour before bedtime (and preferably, not at all).
- **Sleeping pills.** Don't use sleeping pills, melatonin, or other over-the-counter sleep aids. These may be dangerous, and your sleep problems will probably return when you stop using the medicine.
- **Don't drive drowsy.** Teenagers are at the highest risk for falling asleep at the wheel, so don't drive when you haven't gotten enough sleep. Accidents are likely to happen in the middle of the afternoon as well at night.

Appendix G

Resources for Families

RESOURCES

American Academy of Sleep Medicine (AASM)
One Westbrook Corporate Center, Suite 920
Westchester, IL 60154
Telephone: (708) 492-0930
Fax: (708) 492-0943
www.aasmnet.org

Sleep Research Society (SRS)
One Westbrook Corporate Center, Suite 920
Westchester, IL 60154
Telephone: (708) 492-0930
Fax: (708) 492-0943
www.sleepresearchsociety.org

National Sleep Foundation (NSF)
1522 K Street, NW, Suite 500
Washington, DC 20005
Telephone: (202) 341-3471
Fax: (202) 341-3472
www.sleepfoundation.org

Narcolepsy Network Inc.
10921 Reed Hartman Highway
Cincinnati, OH 45242
Telephone: (513) 891-3522
Fax: (513) 891-3836
E-mail: *narnet@aol.com*
www.narcolepsynetwork.org

Restless Legs Syndrome Foundation
819 Second Street S.W.
Rochester, MN 55902-2985
www.rls.org

American Sleep Apnea Association
A.W.A.K.E. Network
1424 K Street, NW, Suite 302
Washington, DC 20005
Telephone: (202) 293-3650
Fax: (202) 293-3656
E-mail: *asaa@sleepapnea.org*
www.sleepapnea.org

National Center on Sleep Disorders Research (NCSDR)
Two Rockledge Center
Suite 7024
6701 Rockledge Drive, MSC 7920
Bethesda, MD 20892-7920
Telephone: (301) 435-0199
Fax: (301) 480-3451
www.nhlbi.nih.govaboutncsdrindex.htm

OTHER ORGANIZATIONS

National Institute of Mental Health (NIMH)
Information Resources and Inquiries Branch
5600 Fishers Lane, Room 15-c-105
Rockville, MD 20807
Telephone: (301) 443-4515
http:gopher.nimh.nih.gov

National Institute of Health (NIH)
Building 1
1 Center Drive
Bethesda, MD 20892
Telephone: (301) 496-4000
www.NIH.gov

American Academy of Pediatrics
141 Northwest Point Boulevard
Elk Grove Village, IL 60007-1098
Telephone: (847) 434-4000
Fax: (847) 434-8000
www.aap.org

US Consumer Product Safety Commission
Office of Information and Public Affairs
Washington, DC 20207-0001
Telephone: (301) 504-0990
Fax: (301) 504-0124 or (301) 504-0025
Toll free consumer hotline: (800) 638-2772
www.cpsc.gov

National SIDS Resource Center
2070 Chain Bridge Road, Suite 450
Vienna, VA 22182
Telephone: (703) 821-8955
Fax: (703) 821-2098
E-mail: *sids@circlesolutions.com*
www.sidscenter.org

SIDS Alliance
1314 Bedford Avenue, Suite 210
Baltimore, MD 21208
Telephone: (410) 653-8226
Fax: (410) 653-8709
www.sidsalliance.org

American Psychological Association
750 First Street, NE
Washington, DC 20002-4242
Telephone: (800) 374-2721 or (202) 336-5500
www.apa.org

PARENTING BOOKS

Children's Sleep

Ferber R. *Solve your child's sleep problems*. New York: Simon & Schuster, 1985.
Mindell JA. *Sleeping through the night: how infants, toddlers, and their parents can get a good night's sleep*. New York: HarperCollins, 1997.
Weissbluth M. *Healthy sleep habits, happy child*. New York: Fawcett Books, 1999.

General Parenting Books

Brazelton TB. *Touchpoints: your child's emotional and behavioral development*. Oxford: Perseus Books, 1994.
Brazelton TB, et al. *Touchpoints three to six: your child's emotional and behavioral development*. Oxford: Perseus Books, 2001.
Clark L. *SOS: Help for parents*. Bowling Green: Parents Press, 1996.
Kranowitz CS. *The out of sync child: recognizing and coping with sensory integration dysfunction*. New York: Berkley Publishing Group, 1998.
Kurcinka MS. *Raising your spirited child: a guide for parents whose child is more intense, sensitive, perceptive, persistent, and energetic*. New York: HarperPerennial, 1992.

Phelan TW. *1-2-3 Magic: effective discipline for children 2–12.* Glen Ellyn, IL: Child Management Inc., 1996.

Adult Sleep

Dement WC. *The promise of sleep: a pioneer in sleep medicine explores the vital connection between health, happiness, and a good night's sleep.* New York: Dell Books, 2000.

Hauri P, Linde S. *No more sleepless nights.* New York: John Wiley & Sons, 1996.

Maas JB. *Power sleep: the revolutionary program that prepares your mind for peak performance.* New York: HarperCollins, 1999.

Walsleben JA. *A woman's guide to sleep: guaranteed solutions for a good night's rest.* New York: Crown Publishing Group, Inc., 2001

Wolfson AR. *The woman's book of sleep: a complete resource guide.* Oakland, CA: New Harbinger Publishers, 2001.

Suggested References

GENERAL REFERENCES

Ferber R, Kryger MH, eds. *Principles and practice of sleep medicine in the child.* Philadelphia: WB Saunders, 1995.

Kryger MH, Roth T, Dement WC, eds. *Principles and practice of sleep medicine.* Philadelphia: WB Saunders, 2000.

Lee-Chiong TL, Sateia MJ, Carskadon MA, eds. *Sleep medicine.* Philadelphia: Lippincott Williams & Wilkins, 2002.

CHAPTER 1: SLEEP IN THE PEDIATRIC PRACTICE

Chervin R, Archbold K, Panahi P, Pituch K. Sleep problems seldom addressed at two general pediatric clinics. *Pediatrics* 2001;107 (6):1375–1380.

Fallone G, Owens JA, Deane J. Sleepiness in children and adolescents: clinical implications. *Sleep Med Rev* 2002;6:287–306.

Owens JA. The practice of pediatric sleep medicine: results of a community survey. *Pediatrics* 2001; 108(3):E51.

Stein M, Mendelsohn J, Obermeyer W, et al. Sleep and behavior problems in school-aged children. *Pediatrics* 2001;107(4):E60.

CHAPTER 2: BIOLOGY OF SLEEP

Anders TF, Sadeh A, Appareddy V. Normal sleep in neonates and children. In: Ferber R, Kryger M, eds. *Principles and practices of sleep medicine in the child.* Philadelphia: WB Saunders, 1995:7–18.

Bonnet MH. Sleep deprivation. In: Kryger MH, Roth T, Dement WC, eds. *Principles and practice of sleep medicine.* Philadelphia: WB Saunders, 2000:53–71.

Carskadon MA, Dement WC. Normal human sleep: an overview. In: Kryger MH, Roth T, Dement WC, eds. *Principles and practice of sleep medicine.* Philadelphia: WB Saunders, 2000:15–25.

Czeisler CA, Khalsa SBS. The human circadian timing system and sleep–wake regulation. In: Kryger MH, Roth T, Dement WC, eds. *Principles and practice of sleep medicine.* Philadelphia: WB Saunders, 2000:353–375.

Dement WC, Vaughan C. *The promise of sleep: a pioneer in sleep medicine explores the vital connection between health, happiness, and a good night's sleep.* New York: Delacorte Press, 1999.

Sheldon SH, Riter S, Detrojan MR. *Atlas of sleep medicine in infants and children.* Armonk, NY: Futura, 1999.

CHAPTER 3: SLEEP IN INFANCY, CHILDHOOD, AND ADOLESCENCE

Carskadon MA, ed. *Adolescent sleep patterns: biological, social, and psychological influences.* Cambridge: Cambridge University Press, 2002.

Mindell JA, Owens JA, Carskadon MA. Developmental features of sleep. *Child Adolesc Psychiatr Clin N Am* 1999;8(4):695–725.

Owens JA, Spirito A, McGuinn M, Nobile C. Sleep habits and sleep disturbance in elementary school-aged children. *J Dev Behav Pediatr* 2000;21(1):27–36.

Sheldon SH. Sleep in infants and children. In: Lee-Chiong TL, Sateia MJ, Carskadon MC, eds. *Sleep medicine.* Philadelphia: Lippincott Williams & Wilkins, 2002:99–103.

CHAPTER 4: EVALUATION OF PEDIATRIC SLEEP DISORDERS

Ferber R. Sleepless in children. In: Ferber R, Kryger M, eds. *Principles and practices of sleep medicine in the child.* Philadelphia: WB Saunders, 1995:79–89.

Sheldon SH Insomnia in children *Curr Treat Options Neurol* 2001;3:1–14.

CHAPTER 6: BEDTIME PROBLEMS
CHAPTER 7: NIGHTWAKINGS

France K, Henderson J, Hudson S. Fact, act, and tact: a three-stage approach to treating the sleep problems of infants and young children in sleep disorders *Child Adolesc Psychiatr Clin N Am* 1996: 581–599.

Goodlin-Jones B, Burnham M, Gaylor E, Anders T. Night waking, sleep–wake organization, and self-soothing in the first year of life. *Dev Behav Pediatr* 2001;22:226–233.

Mindell JA. Empirically supported treatments in pediatric psychology: bedtime refusal and night wakings in young children. *J Pediatr Psychol* 1999;24(6):465–481.

Owens JL, France KG, Wiggs L, Behavioural and cognitive interventions for sleep disorders in infants and children: a review. *Sleep Med Rev* 1999;3: 281–302.

CHAPTER 8: NIGHTTIME FEARS
CHAPTER 9: NIGHTMARES

Krakow B Kellner R, Pathak D. Long term reductions in nightmares treated with imagery rehearsal *Behav Cogn Psychother* 1996;24;135–138.

Mindell JA, Barrett KM. Nightmares and anxiety in elementary-aged children: is there a relationship? *Child Care Health Dev* 2002;28(4):317–322.

Terr L. Nightmares in children. In: Guilleminault C, ed. *Sleep and its disturbances in children.* New York: Raven Press, 1987:231–242.

CHAPTER 10: SLEEPWALKING AND SLEEP TERRORS

Mahowald MW, Schenck CH. Diagnosis and management of parasomnias. *Clin Cornerstone* 2000;2(5): 48–57.

Rosen GM, Ferber R, Mahowald M. Evaluation of parasomnias in children. *Child Adolesc Psychiatr Clin N Am* 1996;5(3)601–616.

CHAPTER 11: HEADBANGING AND BODYROCKING

Dyken ME, Lin-Dyken DC, Yamada T. Diagnosing rhythmic movement disorder with video-polysomnography. *Pediatr Neurol* 1997;16(1):37–41.

CHAPTER 12: BRUXISM

Kato T, Thie NM, Montplaisir JY, Lavigne GJ. Bruxism and orofacial movements during sleep. *Dent Clin N Am* 2001;45(4):657–684.

Nissani M. A bibliographical survey of bruxism with special emphasis on non-traditional treatment modalities. *J Oral Sci.* 2001;43(2):73–83.

Restrepo CC, Alvarez E, Jaramillo C, et al. Effects of psychological techniques on bruxism in children with primary teeth. *J Oral Rehab* 2001;28(4):354–360.

CHAPTER 13: OBSTRUCTIVE SLEEP APNEA AND SLEEP DISORDERED BREATHING

American Thoracic Society. Cardiorespiratory sleep studies in children: establishment of normative data and polysomnographic predictors of morbidity. American Thoracic Society workshop summary. *Am J Respir Crit Care Med* 1999;160:1381–1387.

Chervin R, Archbold K. Hyperactivity and polysomnographic findings in children evaluated for sleep disordered breathing. *Sleep* 2001; 24(3):313–320.

Chervin R, Archbold K, Dillon J, et al. Inattention, hyperactivity and symptoms of sleep-disordered breathing. *Pediatrics* 2002;109:449–456.

Clinical practice guideline: Diagnosis and management of childhood obstructive sleep apnea syndrome. *Pediatrics* 2002;109(4):704–712.

Gozal D, Pope D. Snoring during early childhood and academic performance at ages thirteen to fourteen years. *Pediatrics* 2001;107(6):1394–1399.

Marcus CL. Sleep-disordered breathing in children. *Am J Respir Crit Care Med* 2001;164:16–30.

Marcus CL, Omlin KJ, Basinki DJ, et al. Normal polysomnographic values for children and adolescents. *Am Rev Respir Dis* 1992;146:1235–1239.

Rains JC. Treatment of obstructive sleep apnea in pediatric patients: behavioral intervention for compliance with continuous positive airway pressure *Clin Pediatr* 1995; 34(10): 535–541.

CHAPTER 14: RESTLESS LEGS SYNDROME AND PERIODIC LIMB MOVEMENTS DISORDER

Chervin RD, Archbold KH, Dillon JE, et al. Associations between symptoms of inattention, hyperactivity, restless legs, and periodic leg movements. *Sleep* 2002;25(2):213–218.

Chesson AL Jr, Wise M, Davila D, et al. Practice parameters for the treatment of restless legs syndrome and periodic limb movement disorder. An American Academy of Sleep Medicine Report. Standards of Practice Committee of the American Academy of Sleep Medicine. *Sleep* 1999;22(7):961–968.

Hening W, Allen R, Earley C, et al. The treatment of restless legs syndrome and periodic limb movement disorder. An American Academy of Sleep Medicine review. *Sleep* 1999;22(7):970–999.

Picchietti DL, Underwood DJ, Farris WA, et al. Further studies on periodic limb movement disorder and restless legs syndrome in children with attention-deficit hyperactivity disorder. *Mov Disord* 1999;14(6): 1000–1007.

Picchietti DL, Walters AS. The symptomatology of periodic limb movement disorder. *Sleep* 1996;19(9): 747–748.

Picchietti DL, Walters AS. Moderate to severe periodic limb movement disorder in childhood and adolescence. *Sleep* 1999;22(3):297–300.

CHAPTER 15: NARCOLEPSY

Dahl RE, Holttum J, Trubnick L. A clinical picture of child and adolescent narcolepsy *JAACAP* 1994;33: 834–841.

Littner M, Johnson SF, McCall WV, et al. Practice parameters for the treatment of narcolepsy: an update for 2000. *Sleep* 2001;24(4):451–466.

Wise S. Childhood narcolepsy *Neurology* 1998;50:S37–S42.

CHAPTER 16: DELAYED SLEEP PHASE SYNDROME

Campbell SS, Murphy PJ, van der Heuvel CJ, et al. Etiology and treatment of intrinsic circadian rhythm sleep disorders *Sleep Med Rev* 1999;3:179–200.

Chesson AL Jr, Littner M, Davila D, et al. *Practice parameters for the use of light therapy in the treatment of sleep disorders.* Standards of Practice Committee of the American Academy of Sleep Medicine. *Sleep* 1999;22(5):641–660.

Garcia J, Rosen G, Mahowald M. Circadian rhythms and circadian rhythm disorders in children and adolescents. *Semin Pediatr Neurol.* 2001;8(4):229–240.

CHAPTER 17: INSOMNIA

Chesson A Jr, Hartse K, Anderson WM, et al. Practice parameters for the evaluation of chronic insomnia. An American Academy of Sleep Medicine report. Standards of Practice Committee of the American Academy of Sleep Medicine. *Sleep* 2000;23(2):237–241.

Chesson AL Jr, Anderson WM, Littner M, et al. Practice parameters for the nonpharmacologic treatment of chronic insomnia. An American Academy of Sleep Medicine report. Standards of Practice Committee of the American Academy of Sleep Medicine. *Sleep* 1999;22(8):1128—1133.

Morin CM, Hauri PJ, Espie CA, et al. Nonpharmacologic treatment of chronic insomnia. An American Academy of Sleep Medicine review. *Sleep* 1999;22(8):1134–1156.

CHAPTER 18: INSUFFICIENT SLEEP AND INADEQUATE SLEEP HYGIENE

Carskadon MA, ed. *Adolescent sleep patterns: biological, social, and psychological influences.* Cambridge: Cambridge University Press, 2002.

Dahl RE. The impact of inadequate sleep on children's daytime cognitive function. *Semin Pediatr Neurol* 1996;3:44–50.

Fallone G, Owens JA, Deane J. Sleepiness in children and adolescents: clinical implications. *Sleep Med Rev* 2002;6:287–306.

CHAPTER 19: SLEEP AND MEDICATIONS

Cavallo A, Melatonin: myth vs fact. *Contemp Pediatr* 1997;14:71–84.

Gardiner P and Kemper KJ, Insomnia: herbal and dietary alternatives to counting sheep. *Contemp Pediatr* 2002;19:69–87.

Obermeyer WH, Benca RM. Effects of drugs on sleep. *Neurol Clin* 1996;14:827–840.

Reed MD, Findling RL. Overview of current management of sleep disturbances in children. I. Pharmacotherapy. *Curr Ther Res* 2002;63:B18–B37.

Rosen CL, Owens JA, Scher MS, Gaze DG, Pharmacotherapy for pediatric sleep disturbances: current patterns of use and target populations for controlled clinical trials. *Curr Ther Res* 2002;63:B53–B66.

CHAPTER 20: SLEEP IN SPECIAL NEEDS CHILDREN

Johnson CR Sleep problems in children with mental retardation and autism. *Child Adolesc Psychiatr Clin N Am* 1996;5(3):673–680.

Palm L, Blennow G, Wetterberg L. Long-term melatonin treatment in blind children and young adults with circadian rhythm sleep–wake disturbances. *Dev Med Child Neurol* 1997;39:319–325.

Richdale AL. Sleep problems in autism: prevalence, cause, and intervention. *Dev Med Child Neurol* 1999; 41:60–66.

CHAPTER 21: SLEEP AND MEDICAL DISORDERS

Bloom BJ, Owens JA, McGuinn M, et al. Sleep and its relationship to pain, dysfunction, and disease activity in juvenile rheumatoid arthritis. *J Rheumatol* 2002;29:169–173.

Brown LW. Sleep and epilepsy. *Child Adolesc Psychiatr Clin N Am*1996;5:701–712.

Kirk VG, Morielli A, Brouillette RT. Sleep-disordered breathing in patients with meningomyelocele: the missed diagnosis. *Dev Med Child Neurol* 1999;41:40–43.

Lewin DS, Dahl RE. Importance of sleep in the management of pediatric pain. *J Dev Behav Pediatric* 1999;(20) 4:244–252.

Rose M, Sanford A, Thomas C, Opp MR. Factors altering the sleep of burned children. *Sleep* 2001;24(1): 45–51.

Sadeh A, Horowitz I, Wolach-Benodis L, Wolach B. Sleep and pulmonary function in children with well-controlled, stable asthma. *Sleep* 1998;21:379–384.

Samuels MP, Stebbins VA, Davies SC, et al. Sleep related upper airway obstruction and hypoxaemia in sickle cell disease. *Arch Dis Child* 1992;67:925–929.

Wiggs L and France K Behavioural treatments for sleep problems in children and adolescents with physical illness, psychological problems or intellectual disabilities. *Sleep Med Rev* 2000;4:299–314.

CHAPTER 22: SLEEP AND PSYCHIATRIC DISORDERS

Aronen ET, Paavonen EJ, Fjallberg M, et al. Sleep and psychiatric symptoms in school-aged children. *J Am Acad Child Adolesc Psychiatry* 2000;39:502–508.

Corkum P, Tannock R, Moldofsky H. Sleep disturbances in children with attention-deficit/hyperactivity disorder. *J Am Acad Child Adolesc Psychiatry* 1998;37:637–646.

Dahl RE. The regulation of sleep and arousal: development and psychopathology. *Dev Psychopathol* 1996;8:3–27.

Dahl RE, Ryan ND, Matty MK, et al. Sleep onset abnormalities in depressed adolescents. *Biol Psychiatry* 1996;39:400–410.

Owens JA. Sleep in children with behavioral and psychiatric disorders. In: Lee-Chiong TL, Sateia MJ, Carskadon MC, eds. *Sleep medicine.* Philadelphia: Lippincott Williams & Wilkins, 2002:315–320.

Simonds JF, Parrega H. Sleep behaviors and disorders in children and adolescents evaluated at psychiatric clinics. *J Dev Behav Pediatr*1984;5:6–10.

Subject Index

Page numbers followed by *f* indicate figures. Page numbers followed by *t* indicate tables. *Note:* Medications are listed by generic names.